GOODBYE
AUTOIMMUNE
disease

HOW to PREVENT and REVERSE CHRONIC ILLNESS and
INFLAMMATORY SYMPTOMS using SUPERMARKET FOODS

BROOKE GOLDNER, M.D.

Copyright © 2019
Brooke Goldner, M.D.
Goodbye Autoimmune
GOODBYE AUTOIMMUNE *disease*
HOW to PREVENT and REVERSE CHRONIC ILLNESS and INFLAMMATORY SYMPTOMS using SUPERMARKET FOODS
All rights reserved.

No part of this publication may be reproduced, distributed, or transmitted in any form or by any means, including photocopying, recording, or other electronic or mechanical methods, without the prior written permission of the publisher, except in the case of brief quotations embodied in critical reviews and certain other non-commercial uses permitted by copyright law.

Brooke Goldner, M.D
Published by Express Results, LLC Austin, TX

Printed in the United States of America
First Printing 2019
First Edition 2019
ISBN: 978-1729813904

10 9 8 7 6 5 4 3 2 1

Important Legal Notice And Disclaimer:
This publication is intended to provide educational information with regard to the subject matter covered.
The reader of this course assumes all responsibility for the use of these materials and information Brooke Goldner, M.D. and Express Results, LLC assume no responsibility or liability whatsoever on behalf of any purchaser or reader of these materials.
The methodology, training, products, mentoring, or other teaching does not guarantee success and the results may vary.
The information in this book should not substitute for medical care by a licensed practitioner. Please notify your doctor about any nutritional or alternative therapy you intend to use.

GOODBYE

AUTOIMMUNE

DISEASE

Table of Contents

FOREWORD: By Ellen Jaffe Jones 1
INTRODUCTION: By Brooke Goldner, M.D. 5
Six Steps To Reverse Autoimmune Disease Using Supermarket Foods 9
PART ONE: THE SMOOTHIE SOLUTION 13
Chapter 1: How Do I Get It All In? The Smoothie Solution 15
Chapter 2: Myths About Green Smoothies 19
PART TWO: MINDSET & MOTIVATION 23
Chapter 3: Getting Started 25
Chapter 4: Define & Express Your WHY 27
Chapter 5: Healing Is Love 31
Chapter 6: Letting Go 35
Chapter 7: Forgiveness Part 1: Letting Go of Anger 41
Chapter 8: Forgiveness Part 2: Making Peace With Your Past & Others 43
Chapter 9: Become Unstoppable 47
Chapter 10: Motivation 51
Chapter 11: Be Grateful & Feel Lucky 57
Chapter 12: Conquering Bad Habits To Master Success 60
Chapter 13: Self-Love Meditation 62
PART THREE: HABITS 66
Chapter 14: All About Self Care 68
Chapter 15: Create A Sanctuary 72
Chapter 16: Good Sleep Hygiene 76
Chapter 17: Counting Your Celebrations 80
PART FOUR: ISSUES & SELF-SABOTAGE 84
Chapter 18: Being Good at Healing Makes You Good At Life 86
Chapter 19: Identifying and Eliminating Unsupportive Thoughts 92
Chapter 20: How To Interpret A Bad Day 98
Chapter 21: How To Have Pain Without Suffering 102
Chapter 22: Meditation To Find Limiting Beliefs 104
Chapter 23: You Don't Really See With Your Eyes 110
Chapter 24: Dealing With Cravings 112
Chapter 25: Stop Anxiety Before It Stops You 116
PART FIVE: CASE STUDIES 120
Chapter 26 122

    Case Study #1: Debbie's* Story

        Rheumatoid Arthritis: Going From a Standard American Diet to High Raw Recovery Diet

Chapter 27 126
    Case Study #2: Carla's* Story
        Lupus: Going from a High Starch Low Fat Plant-Based Diet to Full Rapid Recovery Diet

Chapter 28 130
    Case Study #3: Danielle's Story
        Lupus & Sjogren's: From Standard American Diet to Full Rapid Recovery Nutrition Protocol.

Chapter 29 134
    Case Study #4: David's Bridges Story
        Lupus, Scleroderma & Sjogren's: From Highly Processed Standard American Diet to Hyper-Nourishment With Minimal Animal Products.

Chapter 30 142
    Case Study #5: Emily Horowitz's Story
        Sjogren's and Lupus: From "Mostly Vegan" with Expensive Supplements To Rapid Recovery

Chapter 31 146
    Case Study #6: Rachel's Story
        Reversing Lupus & Sjogren's During Pregnancy

Chapter 32 156
    Case Study #7: Meredith's* Story
        A Case of Childhood Lupus

Chapter 33 158
    Case Study #8: Sarah Runco's Story
    Reversing Chronic Pain, Obesity, & Cervical Dysplasia

Chapter 34 162
    Case Study #9: Mary's Story
        Reversing End Stage Kidney Failure from Lupus Nephritis

Chapter 35 166
    Case Study #10: Stacey's* Story
        Lupus & Sjogren's In Six Weeks

Chapter 36 168
    Case Study #11: Karen's Story
        Primary Sjogren's Disease In Six Weeks

Chapter 37 170
    Case Study #12: Mabel's* Story
        Rheumatoid Arthritis Sjogren's & Graves Disease In Six Weeks

Chapter 38 172

Case Study #13: Arthiraani Ramalingam's Story
Hashimoto's Disease In Six Weeks

Chapter 39 176
  Case Study #14: Dawn Ingram's Story
  Rheumatoid Arthritis In Six Weeks

Chapter 40 182
  Case Study #15: Angela's Story
  CREST Syndrome, Scleroderma In Six Weeks

Chapter 41.. 186
  Case Study #16: Genie Holleman's Story
  Lupus & Antiphospholipid Antibodies In Six Weeks

Chapter 42 190
  Case Study #17: Joyce Tompkins' Story
  Sjogren's, Hypothyroid, Myopathy & Peripheral Nervous System Disorder In Six Weeks

Chapter 43 194
  Case Study #18: Mariana Sausedo's Story
  Lupus Cerebritis In Six Weeks

Chapter 44 198
  Case Study #19: Barbara's* Story
  Sjogren's & Lyme In Six Weeks

Chapter 45 202
  Case Study #20: Ashley Lawther's Story
  Goodbye Psoriatic Arthritis

Chapter 46 206
  Case Study #21: Ellen Jaffe Jones Story
  Goodbye Psoriatic Arthritis

Chapter 47 221
  Case Study #22: Rose La Fond's Story
  Hypothyroid, Binge Eating, & Polycystic Ovarian Syndrome In Six Weeks

Chapter 48 225
  Case Study #23: Whitney Lee's Story
  Celiac Disease & Type I Diabetes In Four Weeks

Chapter 49 229
  Case Study #24
  Non-Alcoholic Fatty Liver Disease & Elevated Liver Enzymes

Chapter 50 231
  Case Study #25

PART SIX: FAQ	235
Chapter 51: Frequently Asked Questions	237
CITATIONS	242

FOREWORD
By Ellen Jaffe Jones

**Ny Times Best Selling Author of Eat Vegan for $4 a Day,
2-Time Emmy-Winning TV Investigative Reporter**

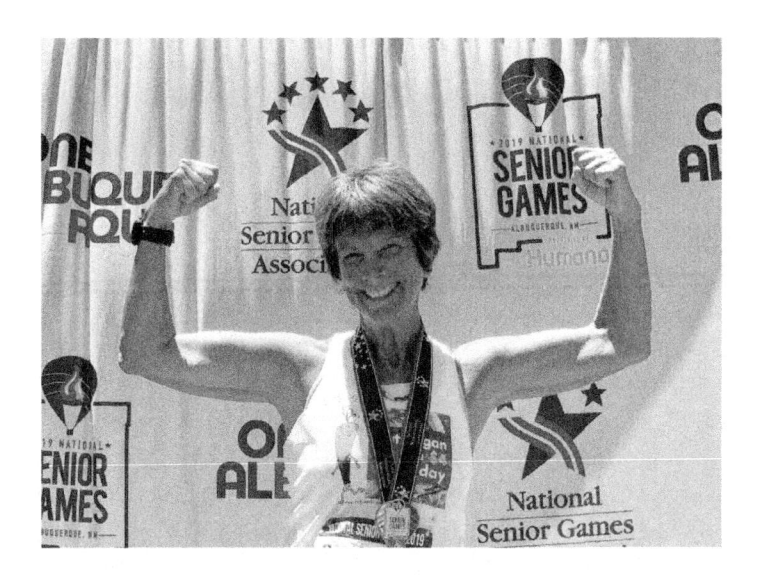

Talk about someone who walks the talk. Dr. Brooke Goldner is the epitome of living by example. It's not enough that she cured her own autoimmune disease when the odds were so against it. She defied all the predictions that she wouldn't make it into adulthood. Dr. Goldner was diagnosed with Systemic Lupus Nephritis with stage IV kidney disease at 16 years old and made a startling recovery from her disease at 28 years old using her protocol, which uses grocery store foods. She has been symptom-free ever since, with normal lab results and no trace of disease in her body. She has been paying it forward ever since.

As a testimonial to her kindness and generosity, she shared groundbreaking results in the incredible and best-selling book, Goodbye Lupus. It has become the go-to resource for many suffering from a variety of autoimmune diseases. It is blissfully simple and easy to follow.

As word spread that her protocol works far beyond lupus for diseases that were thought to be incurable, including a lifetime of excruciating pain and suffering, Dr. Goldner has shared her work and wisdom with the world. She gives endlessly of her time trying to heal those she sees in person and online. She offers free, high-quality content on social media. Many lectures, videos and even free online classes abound.

Dr. G as she is known by her fans, is one of the best, most eloquent and sought after speakers on the lecture circuit today. In her audiences, jaws drop and constant spontaneous applause erupts as slide after slide of before and after photos show dramatic results. Her talks often conclude with an enthusiastic standing ovation.

Beyond the autoimmune diseases that vanish are the "co-morbid" diseases and conditions such as heart disease, diabetes and obesity which often accompany a diagnosis. Those too, often seem to have a way of evaporating. Depression and energy that was sapped are no longer an issue. I know first hand because I too, found myself rapidly spiraling downhill from a genetic autoimmune disease that had no cure. I was depressed and despondent because I was supposed to be the healthy vegan poster child. After following Dr. Goldner's protocol, in just a few short weeks, my condition reversed and I was blown away by the results. A year later, I met Dr. Goldner for the first time on the lecture circuit. I practically jumped into her arms and gave her the biggest hug ever. There's just no substitute for good health. When a doctor gives you your life back, gratitude knows no bounds. Those who have benefited from her work feel this way. Perhaps the most incredible accomplishment is that she achieves this all without any drugs or supplements. All she uses are simple, inexpensive foods you can find at any grocery store. How cool is that?

Dr. Goldner is steeped in results, research and science. While some health care professionals might say that blender drinks are not as good as chewing whole foods, Dr. Goldner says there is no science or study that supports this claim. It takes a high-powered blender full of greens to achieve the results she has attained. Chewing that much in one day is just not possible and smoothies make the blender food-as-medicine go down in the most delightful and easy way. It's the results that count and blood tests never lie.

In her free time, Dr. Goldner has even starred in videos, movies and is an expert for the T. Colin Campbell Center for Nutrition Studies. It is a much shorter list of what she hasn't done.

I, along with thousands of others, are so privileged to have reaped the many benefits of Dr. Goldner's tireless research and work. How she runs all over the world lecturing while having a wonderful, loving family elevates her to wonder woman, rock star status.

As her website says, if you are struggling with illness, weight and/or fatigue and want a healing nutrition plan for chronic illness or weight loss you are looking in the right place.

You could pay a lot of money to go to a retreat, clinic or spa in search of your best health outcomes. But Dr. Goldner's plan is a lot less money and frankly, is so absurdly easy to follow that it is certainly worth a try before anything else. When you read about all the incredible results across many adverse health spectrums in the following pages, you may get chills down your spine and wonder why it took so long to find optimal health. You may also wonder why more doctors don't get a single nutrition class in medical school.

Results are typical. Ask your doctor if plants are right for you. But just make sure your doctor is as educated, trained and results-driven as Dr. Goldner is to create the excellent health that so many of us crave and need.

INTRODUCTION
By Brooke Goldner, M.D.

Having autoimmune disease can take over your life. Chronic pain, lack of energy, and failing organs not only makes you feel awful, but you end up missing out on activities such as work, school, and friendships, because you are sick or too tired to do the things you want to do.

I know all about it. Before I was a doctor, I was a patient. I was diagnosed with lupus at 16 years old. I struggled with kidney failure, arthritis, fatigue, migraines, and even blood clots and mini-strokes over the 12 years I had that diagnosis. I had to take chemotherapy for 2 years and tons of medications, including injecting myself with blood thinners every day. If you read my book Goodbye Lupus, you learned how I changed my diet at 28 years old and the disease completely disappeared. As I am sitting and writing this note to you in 2019, it has been 14 years since I said goodbye to lupus, and I am still healthy and fit. I have been off medications with normal laboratory tests and no symptoms for 14 years! I have also had 2 healthy pregnancies and have the great pleasure of raising two incredibly gifted boys. I also get to look forward to growing old with the man I love; a man who married me when I was sick just hoping to have whatever time he could with me and take care of me as I became disabled, but instead now works side by side with me helping people reverse their diseases and get their lives back. Together we want to give as many people as we can the gift that we got, to live healthy and pain free, to grow old with the person they love, and give back to the world and help others.

I wanted to make sure that everyone had access to the information that saved my life, so I wrote my first book, Goodbye Lupus, in 2015. In the book, I lay out the 6 Steps to Reversing Autoimmune with Supermarket foods in very simple and easy to follow steps that can be taken one at a time, and while many people have read Goodbye Lupus and reversed their diseases and got healthy again, many struggle to take the necessary actions to change their lives. I realized information on what to eat just wasn't enough for most people to change their habits and save their own lives. I needed to help people more.

I decided to retire from my position as a medical director at a nonprofit for homeless and poor youth so I could focus on helping people reverse autoimmune diseases. It was a big pay cut to leave that position, but I did it because I couldn't live with knowing that this information wasn't out there, and that people were dying from diseases I knew how to get rid of. My husband was extremely supportive and encouraged me to do it. We downsized our apartment and eventually moved from California to Texas to decrease expenses so I could start doing this as my primary job without the stress of the high cost of living in California. I started with online video and phone consultations with people and I still do those, and I spend over an hour with people and go through everything they are doing and help them figure out how to do this: I will say "change your breakfast to this, change your lunch to this, oh looks like you're reacting to this food," etc. and I give them a plan. Now some people will follow my instructions and get their health back, and they never need me again. I will get a text message from them a few weeks or months later saying they feel great and a photo of them doing something amazing (and yes, I give every client my cell phone number). The problem was that some people have their appointment with me and then still don't do what I told them to do! I email them my notes and their personalized plan and say "go do this, this is it, this is your personalized plan" and then life gets in the way again and they quit.

So, I said okay, I have got to figure out a way to provide more support and hold people's hands until they cross the finish line, and that's why I created the 4 Week Hyper-Nourishing Rapid Recovery program. Cases in this book come from that plan from people like Carla, Emily, and Rachel. Every person on my 4 Week Rapid Recovery Program gets unlimited access to my cell phone number for the entire 4 weeks for any support they need. It can be menu advice for a restaurant, how to deal with upcoming travel, a wedding, your work schedule, or even a fight with your spouse or your parent if it's creating stress that is interrupting your recovery. Since it is rapid recovery, you are on my most strict form of my diet and I help you every day to make sure you're doing it right and the results are amazing, as you will read about in some of the cases I present here.

The people who have worked on this plan with me have told me it was the best thing they have done for themselves. Eliminating a disease means not only eliminating pain and suffering, but also eliminating medical bills! The issue with the 4-week program is that I can only have 2 people a month on that program because of the intensity of the program and the amount of hours it requires to give that level of care. As I have become more well known, this became an issue, and I knew I had to give the same level of care and contact for more people, and that is why I created the 6 Week Rapid Recovery Group. And I have got to say it's my favorite thing I've ever created. I made it 2 weeks longer than the one-on-one program just in case it took longer to get a group going, and then it was so popular and successful that I kept it that way. I found that in six weeks I can get the same results and often better results than I do with the four weeks one on one. And so, what I could do with the group is get the same results but see more people and if I'm seeing more of you at once, then I can do it for about half the price, so it's more accessible. Helping groups of twenty to thirty people reverse their diseases at a time has given me enormous expertise in the mental and emotional traits and habits of people who succeed with ease, and supporting and transforming the habits of those that struggle to change their diet and their lifestyle. Over time, my group has become not only a place to learn and adhere to the most anti-inflammatory diet possible, but a place to rewire the way people talk to themselves, think about themselves and their illnesses, and learn the habits they need to truly transform their lifestyle so they can successfully reverse their autoimmune diseases and continue to live a healthy life in perpetuity. Graduates of the program tell me they not only feel healthy physically, but they are happy; their anxiety has melted away, and they no longer feel stressed. I want to teach you what I taught them, so you can have those same results.

In this book I will teach you the wealth of knowledge I have accumulated over the past decade on how to successfully change your lifestyle and diet to reverse your autoimmune disease, have optimal health, and enjoy your life. I have seen the major patterns and issues that people struggle with to adopt this new lifestyle, and one of my goals with this book is to give you the lessons and insights I have taught to my clients over the past decade, to help you the reader overcome these issues and have a better chance at success making this your new way of life, and getting back your life.

Every chapter is from the teaching I provide in my 4 Week or 6 Week Rapid Recovery Programs. The focus here is not just on the nutrition but the mindset, the pitfalls, and how to overcome the obstacles and self-sabotage behaviors that might stop you from achieving your goals. There are lessons, meditations, help with limiting beliefs and self-sabotage, and how to create a healing mindset and healing lifestyle. These lessons have helped hundreds of people finally stick with their nutrition, eliminate their stress, and truly nurture themselves in every way to achieve true disease reversal and happier lives. I hope you enjoy the lessons I have taught in my Rapid Recovery program, and that the cases I present here inspire you. I want your story to be the next success story.

SIX STEPS
To Reverse Autoimmune Disease Using Supermarket Foods

The following is a brief review of key points from my book Goodbye Lupus: The 6 Steps to Reverse Disease Using Supermarket foods. To learn this material in depth, I highly suggest you read the book Goodbye Lupus, which contains detailed information and insight to the six steps to healing with supermarket foods, and how this nutrition plan is also supported by the research that has been done in nutrition and disease. It also has my story of how this nutrition protocol reversed Lupus in my body after 12 years of living with chronic illness and gave me extraordinary health and my passion for helping others do the same. You can check out the book Goodbye Lupus on Amazon.com and you can also get more information at http://www.goodbyelupus.com.

Step 1: Eliminate Animal Products

Animal Products include all types of meat like beef, pork, lamb, fish, and chicken. It also includes eggs and dairy products. The reason we must avoid these foods is they contain massive amounts of omega-6 fatty acids, which create inflammation in the body. Eating meat has been shown to increase your risk of all causes of mortality, or death, by 50%![1] Not only are dairy products inflammatory, science shows dairy products cause bone loss, explaining why countries that have the highest rates of dairy consumption also have the highest rates of osteoporosis[2]. Calcium is abundant and easy to absorb from green leafy vegetables like kale and broccoli, without the risks that come with dairy.

Step 2: Eliminate Added Oils

Omega-6 fatty acids are also found in high levels in vegetable oils so they must also be avoided. One of the fastest ways to minimize inflammation and jump-start the healing process, is to eliminate the excess sources of omega-6 fatty acids. Vegetable oils, except for olive oil, are a high source of omega-6 besides animal products already on the "avoid list."[4,8] The more you avoid added oils, the better your cells, organs, and immune system will function. While olive oil is an omega-9 source, they have also shown it to cause damage to the lining of your blood vessels,[3] and since a leading cause of death in people with autoimmune disease is heart attacks, olive oil should be avoided.

Step 3: Eliminate Processed Foods

Processed foods are products containing ingredients that do not occur in nature. People call them foods but they're more like synthesized food-like products. So, what exactly are processed foods? These will be often the items that don't need refrigeration, like chips, processed breads, candy, and sodas. One quick way to find out is to grab a can or box from your kitchen and read the label. If it has a long list of ingredients you cannot pronounce or cannot produce without a lab, it is processed. Processed foods are often full of hidden sugars and oils which further increase inflammation.[5] It has been shown that the body has an inflammatory reaction to processed foods much like having an infection.

We also find trans fats in a lot of processed foods. Food high in trans-fat includes French fries and other fried fast food, some varieties of microwave popcorn, certain margarines and vegetable shortening, packaged cakes and cookies, some pastries, and all processed food that lists partially hydrogenated vegetable oil on the label. These are toxic to your heart and inflammatory.[6,7,9] After eliminating all the foods that cause illness, you may think "now what"? Now, you fill your body with foods that heal you.

Step 4: Hyper-Nourish Yourself with Raw Plant Foods.

Did you know that all of the original medication came from plants? Once scientists figured out how to synthesize these medicines, the pharmaceutical industry was born. While I am a western medical doctor and I believe there is value in prescription medications, which can be life-saving, we must not ignore the natural health-giving medicines that grow on the earth. We don't need to go to the rainforest to get our medicine, we can go to the supermarket and eat foods that flood your body with nutrients to speed up the healing progress. The key to getting the maximal nourishment from plants is eating them raw. That is the best way to get the vitamins, minerals, phyto-enzymes, and phyto-nutrients, which are good plant chemicals. Eat as much greens, raw fruits, and vegetables as you like. The most potent vegetables in terms of nutrient density are dark leafy greens like spinach and cruciferous vegetables like broccoli and kale. Most of your food intake should come from these raw vegetables.

Step 5: Consume Omega-3s Every Day

Omega-3s contain potent anti-inflammatory properties on the cellular level. They are the primary ingredients in the production of your anti-inflammatory immune system.[10] Omega-3 fatty acids are an important part of the membranes of your cells. They become part of the cell phospholipid membrane, which improves cellular function by making the cells more flexible and able to send and receive important messages necessary for basic functions and healing. When your cell membranes are deficient in omega-3s, it makes it difficult for important nutrients to get into the cells, and for toxins to get out. This causes persistence of diseases. Omega-3 fatty acids not only reduce inflammation, they help lower the risk of chronic diseases such as heart disease, cancer, and arthritis. They also regulate blood pressure, blood clotting, glucose tolerance, and nervous system development and functions.[11,12] In addition omega-3 fatty acids are an important part of your brain and nervous system are beneficial for memory, attention, and mood. Omega 3 fatty acids must be eaten to be present in your body, and most people are deficient in omega-3s. The imbalance in omega-3s versus the inflammatory omega-6s is likely one of the main health conditions that causes and perpetuates inflammatory diseases like autoimmune diseases.[12]

Step 6: Water, Water, Water!

Water is essential for most chemical reactions in the body to take place. This means you can have all of the essential ingredients for your health to improve, but without enough water the reactions will not take place or it will be sluggish. There are conflicting arguments about how much water one needs to consume. The FDA recommends eight glasses of water a day (eight ounces each), which equals sixty-four ounces a day, regardless of body size. In my opinion, that is enough to maintain health, but not enough to improve health. What we have found through decades of disease reversal in my clients, is people need a minimum at least ½ of an ounce of water per pound of body weight a day, up to a gallon (128 ounces) of water a day. That means that a person who weighs 150 pounds should have a minimum of 75 to 128 ounces (one gallon) of water a day. A 200 pounds person should have 100 to 128 ounces of water a day. Through repeated trials, we have discovered that that there is a rapid increase in visible results when people consume 96 ounces a day (3 liters), and optimal benefits at 128 ounces (3.8 liters) of water a day for people who are 128lbs or over.

PART ONE
The Smoothie Solution

There is no faster or easier way to eat to heal than by making these green smoothies. You can literally nourish your body and save your life with less than 5 minutes of prep time a day.

Dr. G

Chapter 1
How Do I Get It All In?
The Smoothie Solution

When I first started seeing nutrition clients, I asked them to eat 8 to 10 cups of raw vegetables a day the way I did, focusing on dark leafy greens and cruciferous vegetables. I had them drink omega-3 oils like cold-pressed flax oil to get their omega-3s in. All of that water had to be consumed alone in addition to all the vegetable-chomping they were doing.

While this approach is extremely effective, it only works when people actually do it, and for some people who have never eaten vegetables, especially raw vegetables, this felt like an impossible task.

In 2009, my husband was gifted with a Vitamix blender by a very grateful client who had the body of her dreams thanks to him. We started to play around with it. My husband, who is always looking for ways to simplify and systematize every aspect of his life, had the idea, "what if we blend up all the veggies and drink them?"

At first the result was pretty awful! We just blended up vegetables and drank them and the taste left a lot to be desired. Some combos were undrinkable! Now, you can find a plethora of people sharing what they call "green smoothie recipes" online and in books, but they are usually full of fruit, with just a handful or less of greens. That does make a smoothie that is green in color, but it won't create the rapid disease-reversal that we can achieve when it is made to our standards.

Creating the recipes took some time and testing. The original disease-reversal protocol did not have any fruit, because we found high fruit intake would slow down or sometimes completely inhibit recovery and fat loss. However, we knew fruit could help the flavor, so we ran tests to determine the amount of fruit we could add that would make the smoothies taste good and not affect the recovery rates. Over time and experimentation, we discovered the perfect ratio of vegetables to fruit that creates delicious smoothies that even veggie-phobes will enjoy, and can typically achieve the same health and fitness benefits of vegetables alone. To get these results, make sure the green smoothies have 75% or more (by volume) of packed leafy greens, and 25% or less fruit. When you load up your blender with greens, make sure you push the greens down with your fist or a kitchen tool to get the air out and make sure you truly have 75% of that blender full of packed greens. Then add the flax or chia, and then fill the final 25% of your blender with fruit of your choice. You can use fresh fruit and add ice, or use frozen fruit. The greens must be fresh to get the maximum benefit; nutrients are lost in freezing. I don't mind if the fruits are frozen because we are not using the fruit for the nutrients, we are using them for the flavor.

The smoothies not only make it easier to get all of your raw vegetables in, they also make it easier to get in your omega-3s. You can throw the omega-3 source (flax or chia seeds, or cold-pressed flax or chia oil) right into the blender with the greens and fruit. Flaxseeds and chia seeds are far cheaper than the cold-pressed oils, usually less than $1.50 a pound, and they grind up easily in a high-powered blender like a Vitamix or Blendtec. If you have a lower powered blender, you will want to pulse them with a coffee grinder first. Only grind up how much you plan to use. Do not buy pre-ground of grind them up and store them, since omega-3s oxidize and become inactive quickly when exposed to air. The liquid of the smoothie will protect them from oxidation as you drink it during the course of the day.

The smoothie also simplifies water intake, since a full Vitamix carafe of our green smoothie recipes require about 40 ounces of water to blend. That takes a big chunk out of your water requirements for the day.

The Smoothie Solution is also a big time saver, since you don't need to chop veggies and store them. You also don't need to hunt for an oil-free dressing recipe because no dressing is required! Even more importantly, people love them! The same folks who would balk at a big salad, happily slurp down their smoothies. After all, the only way the veggies, water, and omega-3s will reverse your disease is if you actually consume them, and most people find this is the most convenient and delicious way to hyper-nourish themselves. You get to drink the most anti-inflammatory foods in the supermarket that will give you the health you want, and it takes only 5 minutes a day to prepare them.

The Smoothie Solution has revolutionized our recovery protocol, making eating to reverse your disease or maintain optimal health both convenient and delicious. With a high powered blender, the smoothie also delivers a big hit of energy from all of the vitamins and minerals being released into your system at once. They feel great!

If you are wondering how much smoothie to have, the answer is the more the better, but do as much as you can.

If you are un-used to raw foods, you likely have a slow gut, and fiber will make you bloated and full. While it might be uncomfortable to be bloated, it is not generally something to worry about. Fiber tells your gut to pull water into it, expanding your intestines. If you are drinking 96 to 128 ounces of water a day, you have plenty of water to fill your bowels (and your bladder)! If the bloating is really bothering you, try having small glasses of smoothie spread out throughout the day so your gut has time to process it. Too much at once will make you bloated and gassy. Also, you may benefit from taking a high grade probiotic during your transition into eating raw foods. If you have a lot of gut distress, you can start slow and increase your amounts as tolerated. If you really stick with it, your gut will expand quickly and you will be able to eat far more. For example, in my 6 week rapid recovery group, I start people out on 8 cups of raw leafy greens and cruciferous vegetables a day. Many people feel really full on just that amount, whether it's in smoothies or salads.

If they continue to eat that amount every day, then in a week they can usually increase by another 2 cups a day. At the end of the 6 weeks, many members can eat double the starting amount of raw vegetables and still have an appetite!

Bloating will take time to resolve, and some bloating is normal even with a healthy gut. Remember fiber attracts water, which will swell the intestine, which helps fecal matter move smoothly towards the anus. Imagine a nice lazy river of poop floating towards the exit. Fuller intestines also give the muscles around the intestines something to squeeze during bowel movements, causing much easier and softer bowel movements. This is why people on low fiber diets usually have terrible constipation in addition to terrible health, because the fecal matter is stuck. The answer is not medications, or even powdered fiber, but real fiber rich vegetables and water.

Most people on my plan find they are having bowel movements 3 to 4 times a day, and boy do they feel light and clean! Now on occasion, someone will get constipated on this plan. Why is that? It is because they have such a slow and weak gut that this is more fiber than their gut can handle. The muscle walls are too weak to squeeze that much fiber and water. For those folks I recommend they lower the fiber in the smoothies by using filtered cold-pressed refrigerated flaxseed oil instead of seeds. The filtering removes the fiber from the seeds and the oil lubricates the gut to help things move along more quickly. With severe bloating and constipation, prebiotics and digestive enzymes can be helpful in the early stages as well.

Some people get constipated because they also gave up caffeine when they started rapid recovery. Caffeine is a laxative, so the combination of stopping the laxative of caffeine and increasing fiber can also create constipation. I do not recommend stopping caffeine while increasing your fiber. Make sure there is no dairy or sugar in it though. Then, when your gut adjusts, taper the caffeine. Most people tell me they have so much energy from their smoothies they just don't need caffeine anymore!

Chapter 2
Myths About Green Smoothies

As my hyper-nourishment protocol has grown in popularity, I get more and more emails from people who read or heard that green smoothies are not beneficial or even worse, can be harmful. Here are the most common myths I have come across and the truth of the matter.

1) Green Smoothies will cause weight gain.

I have read posts and blogs created by highly respected doctors in the plant-based world that state this. It really gets me aggravated because it is unscientific, and frankly, dangerous because it warns people off of doing something that can be life-saving for them. They propose that blending greens and fruit will cause a person to have too much sugar at once (from the fruit) and will thereby cause weight gain.

Now, these doctors did not test this theory, nor cite tests or research done in this area. The only things I teach are my results, never my theories, because theories are often wrong, even when created by intelligent people who are right about many other things. In this case, our results prove that people who consume the smoothies the way we prescribe them have rapid fat loss, not fat gain. I agree that a fruit smoothie would not promote fat loss, or a typical green smoothie with mostly fruit, but they do not say that. They generalized and assumed, two very dangerous activities when it comes to giving health advice in my opinion.

My husband, Thomas Tadlock, used to have the largest fitness boot camps in Orange Country California, and he tested the smoothies on his clients, and they had extremely rapid fat loss when they combined the smoothies with his workouts, far faster than they did on low calorie, low carbohydrate or other fad diets. He has also used these smoothies in his celebrity clients to get them fast results that they can sustain. The combination of 75% greens, 25% fruit, flax or chia, and water is not only extremely anti-inflammatory, it is the perfect food for rapid and healthy fat loss.

2) It's better to chew your food versus blend it.

This is another myth often repeated by otherwise well-informed plant-based doctors. I have had the opportunity to change all of their views, but the internet never forgets, and the videos and blogs continue to be shared, and misinformation abounds.

The theory states that since we have enzymes in our saliva that begins the digestive process, we should chew our food up to mix it with our saliva in order to digest the food properly.

There are a lot of faults with this logic. First of all, blending up the greens in the smoothie accelerates the process of breaking down the food and releasing the nutrients so you don't need saliva to start the process. In fact, the blender did a far more efficient job than your teeth would have done with old-fashioned mastication.

The more important reason to ignore this idea, is the fact that people who drink the green smoothies get healthier. As you will see in the case studies in this book, the smoothies do not just make people a little healthier, they have been instrumental in reversing severe chronic inflammatory autoimmune disease, diabetes, and heart disease.

The fact is, this smoothie protocol is reversing diseases faster than any other program that I know of; most people feel dramatically better in a matter of weeks, and many reversing blood markers that have been positive for decades in weeks to a few months. If people were not digesting and absorbing the smoothies, that just wouldn't happen.

Now, if you prefer to eat salads over drinking smoothies, that is totally fine, but there is no reason to do so if you enjoy the smoothies.

I have talked to multiple plant-based doctors who are on the record saying chewing is better, and one of them is now in my Smoothie Shred facebook group, the wife of a second famous plant based doctor called me to ask how much flax to put in his smoothie, and a third has now made videos showing how to make his favorite green smoothie recipes!

The weight of the results has buried the objections, but alas the internet is forever, so it still comes up.

3) Green smoothies cause kidney stones.

This myth has been circulating a lot recently. The premise is that since certain greens are high in something called calcium oxalate, and since the most common type of kidney stones are made of calcium oxalate, then if you eat too much greens, you will get kidney stones. This may sound logical, but this is not the way the body works.

First of all, the most common cause of calcium oxalate kidney stones are dehydration and consuming high amounts of meat.[30] In fact, diets that are high in high fiber vegetables have been shown to decrease the risk of getting kidney stones.[31] Thus, for the vast majority of people, eating high amounts of leafy greens and low amounts of animal protein, will not only reverse chronic diseases, it will protect them from kidney stones.

So where did this idea come from? There are medical problems that can predispose someone to getting calcium oxalate stones even with a plant-based diet.

First, there is a very low percentage of people who have a genetic predisposition to getting kidney stones, that can be exacerbated by eating foods with oxalates in them. This is called Primary Hyperoxaluria. This is an extremely rare genetic disorder of liver metabolism that can result in severe kidney damage. People with this disorder do not produce sufficient amounts of an enzyme that prevents over-production of oxalate (or they do produce the enzyme but it doesn't work properly). While this does make affected individuals predisposed to oxalate stones, it has been shown not to be dose-dependent. This means that someone with this disorder will produce kidney stones, but not because they were eating too much oxalate-rich foods, they would produce oxalate stones even with small amounts of dietary oxalates.

There is also a condition called Secondary Hyperoxaluria, which is caused by excess absorption of oxalate from the gastrointestinal tract due to underlying medical conditions. Usually it is caused by diseases that affect gut absorption, like gastric bypass,[30, 33] Crohn's disease, prolonged antibiotic use,[33] and short bowel syndrome.[30] Some people with systemic disorders like diabetes and primary hyperparathyroidism, gout, and chronic kidney disease with impaired kidney output are also at risk for this condition.[30, 32]

If you have one of these medical issues, it does not mean you can't consume leafy greens, quite the opposite, you need them! You just need to avoid the greens with the highest oxalate content, primarily raw spinach and beet greens. What has worked very well for my clients is simply avoiding spinach, which has far greater oxalate levels than other greens, and using kale instead.

By the way, the information about oxalates is only recently surfacing, and in the meantime, thousands of people have been on the Smoothie Solution over the past decade without a coinciding surge of kidney stones, even in people who have some of these risk factors. If the risk were as high as some propose it to be, I would definitely be the one to observe it, considering how many people I have put on this program. That said, considering there is any increased risk, I would still choose lower oxalate greens if you have these risk factors.

Speaking from a results perspective, I have seen countless miraculous incidences of disease reversal from the green smoothies, but I have not seen proven causes of calcium oxalate stone formation from smoothies. One reason might be that if my clients have significant kidney failure, I always use kale over spinach exclusively because of the lower potassium content, which bypasses the issue completely. The bottom line is that the benefits outweigh any risks by light-years, and of course if you don't blend with spinach often or at all, then you don't need to be concerned.

As a side, if you compare these mild risks to the risk of eating a low fiber diet, or a high animal protein diet, which is causing the majority of diseases people are currently dying from,[1] I believe the conversation about the risks of eating too many vegetables borders on absurd.

PART TWO
MINDSET & MOTIVATION

"If you want to get healthy, you need to be prepared, you need to be motivated, and you need to address the thoughts and beliefs that can steal your motivation and sabotage your success. When you change your mindset to support your best health, the nutrition becomes easy."

Dr. G

Chapter 3
Getting Started

The most important thing you can do to be successful with the healing protocol is to be prepared. That means never leave the house without food. Even with simple errands like running to the gas station or shopping, always bring food with you. You may think you'll just be a couple minutes, but those couple of minutes can turn into a couple hours and now you don't have any food with you. What if you get hungry? You might get tempted and that can snowball into eating the wrong things. People often struggle to make healthy food choices when they are hungry, hence the advice that you should never go the supermarket hungry, because you'll end up with a cart full of things you don't really want to eat! The answer is to always be prepared. Never leave the house without food. It takes some work to make this happen, but you'll be glad you took the extra time to be prepared.

Tip 1 – Invest in a cooler and take it with you when you're driving anywhere. Put a smoothie and other snacks like vegetables and fruits in there along with an ice pack. I used to take a cooler with me to work every day when I worked at the nonprofit. I blended my smoothies beforehand, poured them into jars with ice in them, and put them in a cooler with ice packs to keep them cold. As soon as I got to work, I'd put them in the fridge. I'd drink them all day and didn't even need to take a lunch break. I was prepared. I was also full and energetic all day long.

Tip 2- Buy a large water jug to take with you wherever you go. When I reversed my lupus, I was an intern during my residency. I bought a gallon-sized water container from Walmart with a carrying strap and strapped it over my shoulder and carried it around all day while I rounded in the hospital. It was heavy, and walking up and down stairs with it was good exercise! Because it was literally on my back, I drank it often and finished it with ease. If I had waited for breaks in the day to go get a water bottle or just carried a 20 ounce bottle with me, I would never have gotten all that water in. When it comes to water, I find that people drink however many ounces their water bottle holds. If they have to get up to refill it, water intake goes down.

Tip 3- Buy bulk frozen fruit, fresh bananas, and pre-packaged, pre-washed greens to have on hand for smoothies. At Costco, I can buy large bags of frozen mangoes, pineapples, and cherries that taste great in smoothies. Bananas are best when they have brown spots - that is the perfect time for sweet smoothies. If they are ripe and you are not ready to use them all, just peel them and freeze them for future smoothies. Costco also sells giant bags of power greens (mixed greens like kale and spinach and chard) that are 50% larger than what I can get in supermarkets, enough for 2 blenders. While it is nice to have nice fresh bunches to use for smoothies, washing greens and chopping fruits takes a long time, and if it isn't convenient, then people often quit before they get the results they are after. Note, frozen fruit is ok because we are using them for flavor, not for nutrients. Greens should always be fresh, not frozen.

Tip 4: Experiment with different recipes and flavors for your smoothies. I have a green smoothie recipe book, but I also have free recipes on my website SmoothieShred.com that are simple recipes that just require frozen fruit and leafy greens. They are tried and tested and loved by my family - including my kids.

If you absolutely do not like the flavor of the smoothie you made, don't force yourself to drink it. The last thing you want to do is create an aversion to healing foods. Either pour it out and start over, or if you can't stand to waste it, pour half of the offending smoothies into a jar and then add more greens and different fruits to the remaining mixture to change up the flavor. The best way to disguise flavors is with super ripe bananas, a half of an avocado (takes away the "green taste" or bitterness), or grapes.

You can also take the existing drink and dilute it down with unsweetened almond milk (or cashew milk or coconut milk) which will hide the flavor. You will have more liquid to drink, but it helps disguise the flavor pretty effectively.

Chapter 4
Define & Express Your WHY

The first 2 weeks of changing your diet is the most difficult. First of all, many people who switch from meats, dairy, and processed foods to whole raw plant foods do what we refer to as a detox period. During this time people often feel tired, irritable, achy, or even like they have the flu. Essentially, some people have to feel worse before they feel better. It's difficult to stay motivated under those circumstances if you aren't really focused.

Second, cravings can be very intense in the first 2 weeks, and often peak during the second week. So, you are tired and achy and having intense cravings, which can make you vulnerable to giving up if you aren't truly focused on what you want from your life and why you are doing this.

Now you can understand why people often quit after only 2 weeks when they are trying to do this on their own. That is why one of the first assignments in the 6 Week Rapid Recovery Group is to define your WHY. I define your WHY as your true reason for doing this program: what is the life you truly want that makes doing whatever it takes worthwhile? I write it in all capital letters because it is a big deal that requires big letters!

This is an important assignment that will help you not only get through the first weeks, but get through the program and stay healthy for the rest of your life. Here's what I want you to do: I want you to express your WHY.

What is the reason you're doing the protocol? I don't want you to just address symptoms, like saying "I don't want to have aches and pains" or "I want to have more energy." While these are important issues, they don't really dig deep enough to be considered your WHY. Instead, I want you to think about what you want to happen in your life, because it's the big picture things that motivates us to do something difficult.

I find it is most effective to speak your WHY. There's a power in speaking words out loud. To truly taste the words and feel the vibrations in your throat and your body as you declare your passion and purpose. I encourage you to make a video of yourself so you can watch it and remind yourself every day why you are giving up your food addictions and eating healing foods even though it is inconvenient and difficult to do.

If you aren't comfortable making a video, at minimum write out your WHY and say it out loud to yourself as you write, and read it out loud to yourself every morning.

I also want you to declare your WHY as if it already happened, rather than a wish for what you want to happen. I want you to get used to the feeling of accomplishment that comes from living your best life, and when you say the words as if you already achieved them, it is truly inspiring and motivating. In my group, people will post their WHY videos and cry through them as hope wells up in their hearts. I want you to do the same.

Once you express your WHY, and make it real to you, your motivation skyrockets. Without it, you're likely to be focused on what's going on in your body; the daily aches and pains and struggles. It makes you rely too much on willpower, and unfortunately willpower will often fail. Willpower is about denying yourself what you really want. For example, you know you need your green smoothie, but there is a cookie on the table. When you use willpower, you tell yourself, "I want that cookie but I won't let myself have it". Eventually, you will have that cookie, if not today, then another day when you feel more emotionally vulnerable.

When you use WHY-power, you actually don't want the cookie, because it will rob you of everything you want in this world. It isn't about a green smoothie versus a cookie, it is about my health and happiness and everything I want for my life, versus a cookie. No contest there! When you keep yourself focused on your WHY, the work doesn't seem that hard. This isn't just true for sticking with your nutrition plan, it works for all areas of your life where you are trying to succeed at something very difficult. I did this exercise myself in medical school. My first two years of medical school were so difficult because my joy is helping people. Instead of helping people, the first two years of medical school is all about classes and memorizing textbooks. I'd often read textbooks for 12 hours a day. I couldn't go out often, I was constantly required to study. It's the only time in my life I ever felt depressed. Lupus didn't depress me. Being isolated from people depressed me. One day, I took a lipstick and wrote "Brooke Goldner, MD" on my bathroom mirror, so that every time I looked in the mirror I saw the words under my face.

I felt a surge of excitement every time I saw it. I expressed my why in writing and I made it real to myself. Every time I saw my "why" on my bathroom mirror, I got excited again for medical school and my future. I couldn't wait to get back to hitting the books again. Connecting with WHY I was working so hard, the future I was creating for myself, made the tedious work I faced daily worth every minute. I made my why visible to remind myself that my life was not about studying and reading for 12 hours a day. My life was about what I wanted to do in the world and what I wanted to be in the world. The way we get through things that are hard is by keeping it ever present in our minds, why am I doing this?

I want you to focus on your WHY as soon as you wake up, before you leave your bed. That way when your feet hit the ground, you'll want to go running after that green smoothie because you're so excited about what your life will be like when you are healthy.

After reading this chapter, please complete this assignment so you are ready to get clarity, get excited, and crush this program!

Assignment

There are three parts to this assignment. Say these in the present tense as if you have already achieved your "why."

Step 1: Say in the present tense how do you feel emotionally and in your body. For example, "I feel amazing amounts of energy and joy. I feel my joints and my body moving however I want them to." Talk about how you feel as if you've already achieved your goal and results.

Step 2: Say in the present tense what you are doing. For example, "I'm hiking in the Grand Canyon. I'm running a 5k. I'm running around with my grandchildren." What are you doing?

Step 3: Say in the present tense, who are you inspiring. A lot of us feel even more motivated by doing things for others than we do for ourselves. For those of you who are caretakers and find it difficult to motivate yourself for your own benefit, who are you inspiring? Are you inspiring your kids? Are you inspiring your friends or your neighbors? Are you onstage inspiring rooms full of people who have the illness that you USED to have? Think about it. Who are you inspiring?

Please Complete the WHY assignment before proceeding to Chapter 5

Chapter 5
Healing Is Love

It can be frustrating and scary when you're trying to heal. Eating all these amazing plant-based foods is hard. It's different from your regular diet and routine. It's good for you, but also can make you gassy and bloated. You're missing out on your favorite foods and drinks and cravings can be really strong. You can no longer use food to comfort yourself on a tough day. You are doing something that many people consider weird, and often people who try to convince you not to do it, tempt you to "just have a little" off plan foods, or even try to guilt you into having something that they made for you that is off plan.

It's really hard, and it will also likely be the most important and life-changing thing you've ever done. It can give you the life you've always wanted. It can get you back everything that illness made you lose: energy, vitality, the ability to go out with others or be in the sunlight.

One of the biggest struggles I see, is when people view the healing protocol as punishment. They're upset they're not getting results fast enough, not able to eat what they want, or see others succeeding when they feel like they're failing. Don't compare yourself or your healing journey to anyone else. All of those things hold you back from what you need and from the truth. The truth is healing is love.

Healing is about self-love. It's about learning how to love yourself and your life right now, exactly how you are, to give yourself the serenity and peace and space for the body to heal. It takes a lot of energy and work for your cells to regenerate themselves. It's hard work for your body to create all these new anti-inflammatory immune cells, for those anti-inflammatory immune cells to get rid of the damage from disease, and for those sick cells to dump all the toxins you've been storing all this time. All that takes energy and work for your body. The last thing your body needs is a boss that's high-pressure. A boss (you) that's saying, "hey what are you doing? You're not doing it fast enough. What's wrong with you? I don't even think you know how to do this." Trust me, your body knows what to do. You don't need to second guess it's healing potential. Your body was programmed to heal. Every single cell in your body is designed to heal itself from damage, and if you are chronically ill, it means your body either doesn't have the right tools to do the repair work, or you're continuing to do things to cause continued damage. For most people I meet, it's both. The healing protocol is like doing a lot of renovation work on a house; we need to rebuild broken structures and stop creating more damage to healthy structures.

If you can relate to being a negative boss when it comes to your own recovery, it's time to change your mindset. Realize the voice you hear the most is your own. If you are constantly telling yourself you can't do things, you will make it true, and likely give up. Instead, you need to talk to yourself the way you would talk to anyone else who was suffering, sick, and afraid; you need to be an encouraging and loving voice.

When you feel those worries go through your head, when you question yourself and your body and your ability to get what you want, remember what your body needs most right now is love and understanding from you. Say to yourself: "I love you. That's why I'm giving you the space to do this healing work. I know I've put everyone else before you in the past. I've put you last. I've poisoned you with junk food when what you needed was kale and good things because it made me feel better emotionally. I haven't taken care of you the way I should. Now I will. Now I will give you the space and love you need to do the work you have to do to heal. I won't judge you. I won't pressure you. I won't get mad at you. I'll give you the space you need to heal. I'll give you the love and understanding and healthy foods that I haven't given you until now." Many people feel like their body is their enemy when they are sick, that their body turned against them. It's not your body's fault it got sick. Your body has been fighting for you all along, that is why you are still alive in spite of all the bad food and stress you have exposed it to, because it is still fighting for you. When I realized that it wasn't my body attacking me but instead I was the one attacking my own body with cheese and soda and poor sleep, and that my body was doing everything it could do survive my constant assaults, it changed everything. I realized my body was my best friend, but that I had not been a true friend in return. When I gave myself true nourishment, it quickly eliminated all the diseases I had carried around for 12 years, and I was healthy. And 14 years later, I am still healthy. The path to healing was becoming a nurturing loving friend to my body. You need to do the same.

Your body can heal. Give yourself the space and love and support. Tell yourself you can do this. Be understanding. Be kind. Breathe. Meditate. Listen to beautiful music. Relax. Enjoy friends and nature. Give yourself the time and love and nurturing you truly need. Your body will do the rest. It wants to. It's been waiting for years to heal for you. Healing is truly an act of self-love.

Chapter 6
Letting Go

You might come to realize this is not just a nutrition plan. This is not just a detox for physical health. It's an emotional detox as well. This is a prescription for health for every aspect of your mind, body, and spirit.

After establishing your WHY, the next important assignment is to decide what you're letting go of. In order to create a new life, we must make room for it: new habits, new self-talk, new foods, new feelings.

As time passes, we often accumulate pain. We can be hurt physically through health problems, or mentally and spiritually through emotional abuse and trauma. Sometimes people have hurt for so long, they take on pain as part of their identity. They start to believe, I am wounded, I am defective, I am sick, or I am unworthy. When you create an identity around pain and illness, it is very hard to heal. We don't tend to let go of our identities. That is why I encourage people to work on letting go as an important assignment in the 6 week Rapid Recovery Group as they move through detox and start forming new habits that can heal them. When someone has decided that illness is inherent to their identity, it often shows up through self-sabotage, often unseen by the person doing it. For example, I have seen people who will eat perfectly all day, and then eat a mouthful of off plan food at the end of the day. They will tell themselves, that one bite is no big deal, or that they deserve it for a job well done, or that they still ate better than they used to so it's "good enough". Then they will be confused and upset when they don't have the same rapid results as other members of the group who are doing the plan 100%. In the group I will immediately confront such behavior and ask the person, "What part of you doesn't want to heal? What is good about staying sick?" If you find yourself sabotaging your progress, I encourage you to ask yourself those questions. The answers I have gotten from group members vary; sometimes I find out that they are afraid of getting better because people will expect more from them. They might be expected to work again or go back to school, or take on more responsibilities at home. Sometimes they are afraid that they will give it their all and fail so they hold back. Others feel like illness has become comfortable, it's what they are good at, and they are overwhelmed by needing to change their lives.

When you identify the fears, unsupportive beliefs, and negative self-talk, you can work on these issues to truly recover your health. As a psychiatrist, I specialized in trauma and recovery from unsupportive beliefs, and I am able to quickly help people identify their own self sabotaging thoughts and behaviors so they can start letting go of them and embracing their recovery. I encourage them to understand that not trying and staying sick is worse than trying and failing - after all they still feel like a failure not giving it their all. I help them learn that they don't have to do anything when they get well, that healing is about creating opportunities and possibilities to do what you really want to do, and that you can just say no to things you don't want to do, rather than be too sick to do things. I help them find new passions and hobbies, to feel safe having hope. If you aren't participating in the Rapid Recovery program and you are struggling to overcome these issues, I encourage you to find a therapist who can help you do this, someone who has experience with trauma and cognitive behavioral therapy would be ideal.

So what are you ready to let go of? Is it physical pain? Is it guilt? Is it being less than you can be or putting yourself in the shadows? Is it being overweight? Is it being a sick person? Is it stopping yourself or letting yourself down? Is it putting yourself last? What is it you have taken on that you're willing to let go of?

Until you let go of whatever that is, consciously and in a committed way, there's a part of you that will resist getting better. If you don't let go, it stays a part of your identity. If you've incorporated into your identity you are sick, that you are defective, that you are an overweight person, that you're an unworthy person, then you either won't get healthy, or you will find a way to backslide back into old habits after you do experience recovery. Just like I asked you to find your WHY, now I want you to write what you're letting go of.

I once taught at an event for people who want more happiness and success, where they made attendees do an exercise in letting go. Everyone sat around a fire across from a huge lake and wrote down on a piece of paper what they were letting go of. Then each person walked out to the lake and yelled it as loud as we could with all of their intention, "I am letting go of" followed by whatever the thing was that they were letting go of. After they screamed it loud into the night, they burned it in the fire. It was a euphoric feeling for people, they looked happy and excited. I want that feeling for you too. You don't have to scream it into your neighborhood and have the neighbors call the police, but I want you to write what you're letting go of. I want you to speak it out loud. "I am letting go of chronic pain." "I am letting go of being second-best." "I'm letting go of putting myself last." Whatever it is you feel that has become part of the identity that might be holding you back, write it down and then say it out loud.

Don't write the first thing that pops into your head. Sit and close your eyes and meditate on it. What have I been carrying with me? What have I accepted into my identity that is sick? What am I carrying around with me that is part of my identity as a sick person? Whether it's emotionally, psychologically, or physically, decide what you need to let go of. Think about it. Mull it over. Be brave! Share it, so you can release it and get it out of you.

For me, one thing I needed to let go of was chronic pain. Even though I was completely healed, I continued to carry pain in my neck and shoulders. I blamed it on reading all the time or traveling all the time. I went to masseuses and chiropractors and no one could help, at least not for long. It seemed like nothing worked to relieve the pain in my neck and shoulders. I had an incredible conversation with some friends, and I realized there might be a part of me that was holding on to chronic pain. I asked myself why would I hold on to pain when I don't need to? What does having this mean to me? I was surprised by the answers. The first answer I thought of, was that the pain is a way to relate to people who are suffering. I breathed through that thought, and the next deeper thought was that my neck pain was where I carried my guilt for not being able to do everything for everybody else. I realized that I had a belief that I needed to take care of everyone and make sure that they felt ok, and that I thought was letting people down by not being there for everyone in my family all the time, especially once I had my own children. I had to face I couldn't fix everyone, and that people all need to learn to take care of themselves and not just rely on me. I realized that I don't need to carry that pain with me. I am doing everything I can as a human being. I am empathic and compassionate and I don't need pain to connect with others. I also had to be okay with the fact I can't do everything or be everything to everyone. When I released myself from all of that responsibility, I immediately felt the pain leave my shoulders. It was miraculous. Whenever I felt the pain creeping back, I reminded myself that I don't need it, and I felt relief.

Now that neck pain was not inflammatory, but for inflammatory pain, it works the same way: research has shown that stress and depression are inflammatory in the body, so the more you talk negatively to yourself, the more literal illness and pain you have in your body. This is not New Age ideology but actual science. If you want to help your body heal, you need to work on the mindset and self-talk, you need to let go of the negative unsupportive beliefs and allow hope to enter.

We often carry pain physically that is connected to our emotional being and illnesses. When we carry pain every day, part of us decides that's who we are and what we deserve. Give yourself permission to let go. Become the person you're meant to be. Have the most amazing life you're meant to have by letting go.

After reading this chapter, please complete this assignment so you are ready to let go of negativity and self-sabotage and truly embrace your new healthy body and life!

Assignment:

Step 1: Sit in a quiet space and ask yourself, "What do I do that keeps me sick?" "What do I tell myself that makes me want to give up or quit?" "What is scary about getting better?" "What is scary about trying?" Really sit with the questions, think about how you talk to yourself and how you treat yourself. What thoughts and behaviors are you ready to let go of?

Step 2: Write down what you are letting go of. Let it flow. Fill up the page and breathe; feel yourself getting lighter as you let go. Speak the words out loud after you write them and declare your intention to let go.

Step 3: Every time you find yourself slowing down or going back to negative habits or self-talk, reread your letting go assignment, add to it if necessary, then go back and read your WHY out loud again and recommit to yourself.

Please Complete the Letting Go assignment before proceeding to Chapter 7

Chapter 7
Forgiveness Part 1: Letting Go of Anger

Out of all the emotions we experience, anger is by far the most debilitating. Once anger catches hold of our life, it takes us in a downward spiral. It can ruin our life. People hold on to anger because they believe being angry at some person who did something a long time ago somehow punishes the other person. It never works that way. It's almost like people believing that if they take some poison and drink it themselves, the person they're mad at will die. It just doesn't work that way. It only ruins your life, not theirs. You're the one who feels the negative effects, not the other person you're angry with. That's why it's important to figure out a way to let anger go.

In order for anger to leave your body, especially if it's a deep hurt, you've got to relive the experience and resolve the deep down inside physical, mental, and emotional pain. Tell the person how you felt in a way where you understand that they get it. Now, you don't actually need to tell them in reality or in person, you can do the following assignment and visualize the communication, and we have found that people find this just as satisfying. After that, you can have peace inside. You said what you needed to say. There's a balance inside your own universe. You can move on. That's what letting it go means. You let it go so it doesn't come up for you anymore. Anger is not something you forget. If someone does something horrible to you, you don't forget, but out of necessity, forgive. That way you let it go, it doesn't get brought up in your mind, body, or spirit, things don't remind you of it anymore and you live a much happier life.

This next exercise will help you let go of your anger. It's not an easy exercise, but it's one of the greatest exercises you can do for yourself and your overall health. Think of one person you are angry at. It can be recent. Think of someone or a group of people you got upset and angry about. I want you to picture that person in a chair sitting in front of you right now. I want you to imagine them listening to you with complete undivided attention. I want you to imagine them listening to you explain to them that what they did to you hurt you very much.

Then, I want you to picture them telling you how sorry they are for what they did to you. I want you to hear them say they're sorry, and that they would never ever had done what they did had they known it caused you so much pain or affected your life this much. Hear them explaining to you that they only did what they did out of reaction to their own past issues and personal beliefs. They wouldn't have done the things that hurt you if they realized how much pain it caused you. Then I want you to picture yourself telling them, you forgive them. If you're not willing to forgive just yet, at least say you're willing to let it go. Picture yourself reaching over and hugging that person. If you can't go that far, shake their hand and tell them either you forgive them or you're willing to let it go.

Now, bring this image closer to you as if it's happening in real life. Take a deep breath. On the exhale, relax and let it go. Put a big smile on your face. Forgiveness is the magic key. Remember everyone, including yourself, does the best they can at the time with their own beliefs, past histories, and personal traumas. Everyone's always trying to do the best they can. When you forgive, you forgive them for you, so you can stop hurting, not for them.

The idea behind this exercise is you get this communication out in your own head. Expect nothing from them if you ever confront them for real. It's not about them. It's not for them. Don't expect the sorry. Don't even expect them to pick up the phone if you call them. It doesn't matter. You forgive them for you. Once you release that person you're angry with from their deed, you release yourself from all the negative energy around that deed. You can use that new space and new light to move on in your life. You get the abundance and happiness you deserve. Start with one person. Do you feel lighter from forgiving? You deserve your "day in court" so to speak.

You deserve to say to that person what they did to you and how it affected your life. This is your chance. The beauty is it's in your mind. It doesn't matter if the forgiveness happened in your mind or in real life. To the brain, it's all the same.

Chapter 8
Forgiveness Part 2: Making Peace With Your Past & Others

For many people, forgiveness is a vital part of letting go of past pain. When people are trying to let go of illness and pain, a lot of times I find folks store emotional pain in their bodies. It makes sense if you think about it. We know that anxiety, depression, and stress is inflammatory in the body. If you haven't released the emotional pain, you can't release the physical pain that goes with it. A lot of emotional pain comes from holding on to anger and holding on to hurt. The next step in healing is to work on embracing forgiveness so you can let go of the pain and stop the cycle of inflammation that it causes. Once you express and release the anger the way I taught you to in chapter 5, the next step is letting go of the pain behind the anger.

Think about who you are forgiving. What pain are you willing to let go of? If you don't forgive, you hold on to that pain in your body forever. If somebody hurt you, holding on to anger allows that person to continue to hurt you every single day. If you don't want to let that person hurt you anymore, you need to forgive. Forgiveness doesn't mean you're saying what they did is okay.

Forgiveness is saying I will not carry the pain from what you did with me anymore. You can forgive someone you love, someone you hate, or you can forgive yourself. Forgive as much as you can. Let go of the hurt and anger so you can heal. It's about you.

Forgiveness is something many people struggle with. People often tell me that they feel like forgiving a person means they are condoning what they did, like we let them off the hook. You may feel as if you are saying, yes, it's fine you hurt me or I allow people to hurt me. The truth is, you holding on to anger and hurt about something someone else did does not hurt the other person at all. They don't feel your pain. When you forgive, you are saying "I won't let you hurt me anymore. I won't let you steal my health or happiness." We don't forgive to help somebody else feel better. We forgive so we can move on. When we hold on to anger, we are putting ourselves in prison. We are not letting ourselves have the happiness we want. If someone hurts you, wouldn't the best revenge be to overcome it and enjoy your life again?

One person who opened my eyes to the power of forgiveness is Keith Leon. He's a motivational speaker and author. His sister's boyfriend murdered her. Keith was able forgive the boyfriend for killing his sister. When asked, how do you forgive something so heinous? He said that when he learned what happened, his first though was that he wanted to kill the boyfriend. Then he realized that if he could have that thought, he could be capable of murder, which made them alike. He realized if he lived the life that that man lived, he could have done something that terrible as well. He realized that all of us have the same ability to act that way under the right circumstances and he forgave him for being a broken human who had a terrible life. The pain he experienced losing his sister was bad enough, he decided that he didn't need to hold on to the anger too. He is a loving and sweet man who gives a lot of people guidance and peace and his story is inspiring. I have also watched powerful forgiveness stories online, like a Holocaust survivor meeting and forgiving a Nazi soldier, so she could let go of the pain of the war. The ex-soldier broke down crying. When we forgive, we do not condone or encourage bad behavior, we just release the pain and suffering and embrace our own happiness and peace. Forgiveness is such a powerful tool.

There's a cool story about the power of forgiveness called "Parable Of The Little Soul" by Neil Donald Walsch. It's helped me and others. I hope it helps you too.

"There was once a little soul who knew itself to be light. This was a new soul and so eager for experience. I am light, it said, I am the light. Yet, all the knowing of it and all the saying of it could not substitute for the experience of it, and in the realm from which the soul emerged there was nothing but light. Every soul was grand, every soul is magnificent, every soul shone with the same brilliance of awesome light. And so, the little soul in question was as a handle in the Sun. In the midst of the grandest light of which it was a part it could not see itself nor experience itself as it truly was. Now, it came to pass that the little soul yearned and yearned to know itself, and so great was its yearning that one day I said, so God said, do you know little one what you must do to satisfy this yearning of yours? Oh, what god I'll do anything, the little soul said. You must separate yourself from the rest of us and then you must call yourself upon the darkness. You may choose to be any part of God you wish to be, I said to the little soul.

You're the absolute divinity experiencing itself, what aspect of the divinity do you want to wish to experience as you? You mean I have a choice, said the little soul. I answered yes you may choose to experience any part of the divinity through you.

Okay, the little soul said. Then I choose forgiveness. I want to experience myself as the aspect of God called complete forgiveness. Well this created a little challenge as you can imagine, there was no one to forgive. All I have created is perfection and love. No one to forgive, said the little soul incredulously. No one, I repeated. Look around you, do you see any souls less perfect less wonderful than you? As the little soul twirled around it was surprised to see itself surrounded by all the souls in heaven, they were all light. I see none less perfect than I, who shall I be able to forgive? Just then another soul stepped forward from the crowd, "you may forgive me", said the friendly soul. "For what," asked the little soul. "I will come into your next physical lifetime and do something terrible to you so that you have the opportunity to forgive." "You would do that, being such a perfect light, you would do something terrible just so I could know myself as forgiveness?" "Yes, I would do that for you," he said. "But how will you know what to do," asked the little soul. "Well I'll think of something but I need a favor from you. Because in order for me to do this terrible thing, this terrible thing to you that will make you able to forgive me, I will forget myself, I will forget that I am light. So, what I need for you is one thing." And the little soul said, "anything, I'll do anything to experience myself as forgiveness." He said, "I need you to remind me of who I am when I become so dark that I'm able to hurt you, I'll need you to remind me that I am light, and through your forgiveness I can heal as well."

I think that is such a beautiful story. In order for any of us to do something awful, we have to forget we were born perfect and beautiful and light. We become darker and darker when others hurt us, and more capable of hurting others as well. I think it helps if you think of the person who hurt you as someone who is not evil or awful but someone who forgot themselves. You don't need to hate them. You need to find love in your heart so they can also remember who they are. We don't need to carry around the pain other people have given us. Physical pain, that's easy. Emotional pain is harder. When we see the other person as just someone who's lost in the darkness, we can forgive. Not only for them, but for us. We don't need to carry that pain forever. Anger and holding on to pain is how people continue to hurt us. To end all that, forgive.

Who are you forgiving? What pain are you willing to let go of? Now is your time to heal. I know you can do it. Just breathe. You can do this.

Chapter 9
Become Unstoppable

I hope you're seeing how focusing on your WHY, letting go, and forgiveness creates space in your heart and in your life for healing and happiness. The next exercise is learning how to become unstoppable. For this assignment, I want you to look within. There are times as you start the healing protocol or another project that was important to you where you may have had thoughts or habits or behaviors, judgments, or feelings that stopped you or took you off course and away from being successful. I don't want those thoughts, behaviors, emotions, or habits to ever stop you again. That's where becoming unstoppable comes in.

I want you to sit in reflection and think. When have I eaten foods that are unhealthy and off-protocol? When have I just not met my minimums? When have I have not done my self-care? What are the reasons I've given for not doing my self-care or exercise? What are the thoughts, behaviors, and habits stopping me from doing this healing protocol 100%? What has stopped me over the past weeks or right now? If you haven't started yet, look at other times you tried and did not succeed at something you really wanted to do and look at what you said to yourself or did that got in your way. I want you to write those down. Write the thoughts, behaviors, and habits that got in your way. Then I want you to create a plan for how you'll never let those habits stop you again. That's called becoming unstoppable.

Look at yourself. What are the excuses I've given? What are the things I've told myself were the reasons I can't do things? What are the emotional events I've used as a reason not to care for myself, either through my nutrition or exercising self-care? After you've looked at yourself, say to yourself, "here's my plan to never let those things happen again". Whether it's a plan to be more regimented in your schedule so you never think you're out of time, or it's a plan to make meditation something you do when you first wake up every morning so you can't say you don't have time to do it, make a plan and put it into action. If you realize you need to work with a therapist to overcome some traumas and emotional blockages you felt stopped you from embracing the protocol, then give yourself the counseling you need. Remember when you're depressed or anxious you create inflammation. Great planning and the right support will overcome bad habits, so write down your plan and your schedule and stick it. Notice thoughts that say you can't or you shouldn't if they come up, just notice them, and then just keep taking action anyway. In our Rapid Recovery Group, we often help people with noticing their sabotaging thoughts and just letting them go and act anyway. Examples are people who decide not to drink all of their water because they are driving and don't want to stop, or they are short on their food because they forgot their food when they went out. I help them see that your body doesn't understand your reasons or excuses, you either gave your body what it needs to heal or you didn't. You are healing or you aren't. Instead of deciding why you can't do something, plan on how you WILL do it, even if it's inconvenient, because your health is all that matters.

Assignment:

Sit down and think about the reasons you have either eaten off plan, not met the minimum guidelines, or did not take care of your body with proper sleep or self-care. Write down what stopped you or threatened to stop you? What did you tell yourself that made it ok to behave in a way that hurt your health? What excuses or reasons did you give?

Then write down your plan to never let any thought or reason or excuse ever stop you again. If you've overcome these roadblocks in other areas of your life, what techniques are working for you? Keep all the skills that work for you, plan around obstacles, and put yourself as your first priority. Become unstoppable

Complete the Become Unstoppable assignment before proceeding to Chapter 10

Chapter 10
Motivation

Motivation is important when making a life changing decision such as following the Rapid Recovery Nutrition Protocol. Sometimes when folks are not doing what they need to do, they say they're not motivated. I don't think that's ever the case. We're always motivated. We're either motivated to do something or we're motivated not to do something. Sometimes we feel motivated to do something and not do something at the same time, that's called ambivalence. When you have ambivalence, you are frozen and tend not to do anything. If there's part of you that wants to and a part of you that doesn't, it's easier not to do anything, right? That's how many people feel about eating. There's part of me that's heard vegetables are good for me but then I heard some study that spinach might cause problems. Maybe I won't eat vegetables because of it.

That feeling of being unsure because both sides seem legitimate is called ambivalence. Besides ambivalence, there's also polarizing motivation. Polarizing motivation is when you want to succeed and part of you wants to fail at the same time. When you've got a part of you that's scared or feels you don't deserve success and healing, you will do things to sabotage yourself. Often it will be so subtle you won't even know you're doing it. Being short two ounces of water sounds okay, but it's not. The minimum is 96 ounces because that is the minimum amount of water intake that has brought about full disease reversal in my program. Less than that, below the minimum, would therefore stop you from getting that result even if everything else is done right. I also see people eat 100% on plan all day, and then "reward" themselves with a piece of milk chocolate or eat a bite of off-plan food, and then tell themselves it's ok because everything else was on plan. When you take a step back away from the excuses and just look at the results, you can see that all the eating on protocol is aligned with the part of them that wants to get healthy, and that piece of chocolate or that bite of chicken is the part of them that wants to stay sick. Now, people rarely want to stay sick consciously, it is their unconscious fears and doubts that drive the self-sabotage behavior. In my Rapid Recovery Group, I have people really evaluate the circumstances that led to either eating off plan or letting themselves fall short; the thoughts and feelings leading up to taking those actions. While they initially will try to make it seem like no big deal and say "I'll do better next time," I don't let them get away with that because if we don't find the real reason it will happen again. When we dig deeper then we find the truth; that the person felt depressed and thought the chocolate would be comforting, or the person has a belief that she is a failure and unconsciously sabotages herself to make the belief come true. When we uncover the real thoughts and beliefs that drive the behaviors, we can truly change their lives. When you recognize the thoughts and decide to take action for your health in spite of them, you will win back your health and have a much happier life.

There's no "almost" for reversing disease. You're either doing what it takes to recover your health or you're not. While you can get better with each thing you add to your life, to fully recover your health, you need to commit 100% to your recovery. You want to make sure everything you're doing is fully aligned with your recovery and you are not holding back at all. I don't want you to hold back. I want you to win. I want you to be successful. I want this to be your last stop for your health. From here on out, your whole life is now new and wonderful and positive and exciting because of the work you did following the protocol.

So, what do you do if you fall off the plan - either holding back or eating off plan?

The first thing you need to do is acknowledge it. Acknowledge there's a part of you not motivated to move forward. That's what that is. Imagine it this way: you're riding a go-kart but you keep your foot dragging on the ground. You're moving forward but you're dragging your foot trying to slow down the progress. Ask yourself what part of me doesn't want to get better? What's good about staying the way I am? What's good about staying sick? There's always something good about staying the same. There's a reason people stay in a bad situation, whether it's a bad relationship with a person or bad relationship with food. There is always something positive about it. It might be that it's just what you are used to and something new is scary. It might be that you are afraid of failing so not really trying seems like it will hurt less. It might be what I named Wounded Overachiever Syndrome, when you were once a perfectionist who did everything for everyone, but then you got sick and couldn't do anything anymore, and now you are afraid to try. Sometimes it's just that it's comfortable and your current normal, even though you hate it. One client said, "I'm good at being sick. I know how to do this. I know how to be sick. I don't know how to be healthy. I'm afraid that if I'm healthy, people will ask me to do things. If I'm healthy, I won't have an excuse to say no." Do you feel that way? Or maybe you're worried that if you do more, people will have more expectations, and you'll relapse and let everyone down. Even when there's a negative situation, there's always a positive aspect to it, and that is ok.

Here's the truth: if you are super healthy and someone invites you to do something, you can say no. You don't need to be sick to say no. People still love us even if we say no. Be honest. You'll always have the opportunity to say no. Nothing bad will happen to you because you're doing everything to take care of yourself. Acknowledge this and let it go. Being healthy means you can choose what you want to do instead of being forced to say no to things because you can't. Therefore, health gives you options and power.

Another client did amazing the first six weeks of the protocol but then went back to eating badly. She made herself sick again. When I asked 'why?' she didn't know. That's what we worked on for the second round – finding out why she truly stopped taking care of herself so she could focus on really letting it go. When we dove into her thoughts and the emotional work, she realized that deep down she felt she didn't deserve to be healthy. During her childhood experiences she developed a belief that she was unworthy. So, while she was committed and followed the plan while she was in the Rapid Recovery Group and had amazing results, when she graduated feeling energetic, positive, and pain free, that part of her that thought she shouldn't have healing in her life sabotaged her motivation and she let the unhealthy foods creep back in and make her sick. On her second round in the group we confronted those thoughts and developed healthier beliefs about herself. She decided she really does deserve to be healthy. Now she knows her triggers for self-sabotage, she can recognize the thoughts and cut them off before she acts on them. Since she has decided she deserves to be healthy, she won't pick the wrong foods and sabotage herself again.

I had another client who was getting better in the healing protocol 6 week rapid healing program and then went really off. She went from raw foods to chips and sodas. She felt depressed and angry at herself, which only made her want to keep eating badly. I validated her feelings and gently asked her "what part of you wants to be sick?" She dug deep and realized it was because all of her siblings have diseases. All of them are ill but she was the only one to embrace nutrition for her recovery. She was the only one getting better while the rest of them got sicker, and she felt guilty. Why does she get to be better while all of them are sick? She had to acknowledge these thoughts and feelings and then let go of the guilt and feeling like she doesn't deserve to get healthy while her siblings are still suffering. She needed to ask herself "Do I deserve to be healthy even if other people don't make the same choice?" The answer is yes. She also realized that her recovery could inspire her siblings to try what she did, and if not them, she could help others who are open to learning and trying.

Another example is a client who was going off plan because she told herself she deserved a treat. She would eat perfectly all day and then have a cookie or glass of wine at night. We talked about how being healthy is a treat, not being sick. She later acknowledged that being sick was a way of punishing her family for not supporting her. When she was sick, they didn't believe her. She felt if she got healthy, it would let them off the hook. That's a powerful thing to realize about yourself and your motivation.

If you're struggling that's okay. It just means you have mixed motivation. The program itself is simple in terms of execution. It takes five minutes to make a smoothie or fill up your water bottle. You can take fifteen minutes to meditate or relax. You don't even have to do fifteen minutes at once, you can do five minutes 3 times a day or 3 minutes five times a day. There's 1440 minutes in a day and most people only sleep for 420 minutes, so that is over 1000 minutes left! The protocol has basic requirements. If you're finding it hard to follow, there's a part of you fighting against it. Once you're honest with yourself, you can tell yourself, it's okay to be afraid but I will do the protocol anyway. It's okay to feel guilty but I will do the protocol anyway. It's okay to have cravings or be tired or cranky at first, but I will do the protocol. Stop finding reasons to stop or quit and instead focus on your WHY and why you will not let yourself down. If you can't do it on your own, get more support. We spend countless time in the Rapid Recovery Group helping people overcome these limiting beliefs and behaviors. We can do that effectively because of my training as a psychiatrist, and because my husband Thomas, who co-runs the group, is a personal development guru who teaches people the success mindset; helping people overcome limiting beliefs and behaviors so they can have the life they want. Because of this we are good at helping people identify and extinguish what is often unconscious beliefs causing their self-sabotage behaviors. If you are struggling with motivation and you don't know why or how to stop, you want to have professionals who understand the mind and motivation on your side to help you overcome these difficult issues.

You're not just healing your body, but your mind and spirit too. The more you can get this aligned with what you want, the faster all of this will heal. You deserve to be healthy.

Chapter 11
Be Grateful & Feel Lucky

A week after we moved to Houston, Hurricane Harvey arrived and brought massive floods. Our street had over five feet of water! It looked like we lived on a lake. Our house happens to be the highest point on our cul-de-sac and while all of our neighbors' houses were deluged with water, the floods came to our house and stopped at our front doorstep. It flooded all the other houses in our street. Our neighbors across the street got four feet of water on their first floor. The water was literally 3 inches away from going over our front step into our house and the rain just stopped. It was extraordinary. Now, most people would agree that was very lucky, and I think so too. Here is the secret to my happiness though, no matter what happens to me, I have already decided that I will be okay. If the water had come and flooded our house, I would have been okay. If we had to be rescued by boat, I would have been okay. If I had to wait out the storm in a shelter, I would have been okay. Whenever storms hit, whether it be an autoimmune disease or a hurricane, you need to tell yourself you'll be okay.

Storms will always come, we can't control the weather. What we can control is how we react. We can weather the storms and we don't have to suffer. There's a difference between bad things happening and suffering. While we can't prevent bad things from happening, suffering is always a choice. I remember when I did two years of chemotherapy for my failing kidneys from age 16 to 18. My friends were going to the beach, having fun, and I was home throwing up. Even as I laid on my bed watching Three's Company reruns and drinking club soda trying not to vomit, I felt lucky. I didn't feel lucky that I had to take chemo, but I felt lucky I wasn't dead. I felt lucky I didn't have something worse. I felt lucky I wasn't disabled. I felt lucky that I had an amazing family that loved me. At the end of each day, even at 16, I would think no matter what I need to deal with, I would never trade my life for anyone else's. I feel lucky to be me. I got upset, but I let it fall away. I expressed it, I cried about it, and then I said "I'm still okay." I'm not dead. I will keep living. I'm still here and am grateful for my life. I can learn and I can enjoy my life and I can help others and life is worth living. So, on good days I read my textbooks or visited friends and enjoyed my family. And on sick days I took my medicines and I rested.

My grandparents on my mother's side are Holocaust survivors who immigrated to the United States after World War II ended. They had lost brothers and sisters and parents and grandparents between them to senseless murder. They had barely survived themselves. They had run from Poland to Russia, and instead of being trapped and tortured at Auschwitz or Lodge with their family, they were starving in a work camp in Siberia. In spite of everything they endured, they both were happy people, who told me that "every day you wake up is a good day". My grandmother, even as an old lady, used to smile at her family and say "I'm a lucky girl!". I took that to heart; I was free and loved and that was enough to feel lucky.

When I got to medical school I relapsed and ended up having mini-strokes from blood clots caused by anti-phospholipid antibodies from the lupus. I was scared and upset when this happened, I was so close to living my dream of becoming a doctor in spite of everything I had lived though, and now my life was in danger again. I cried about having to inject myself with blood thinners every day from now until forever (according to my doctors), and that I could have a stroke that could end my life or take away my brain, the one organ that got me through every ordeal I had with lupus. When the tears dried, and yes you should cry until you are done, I remembered that I was going to be okay. I was still alive. I did not have a massive stroke. I had a new medicine that would thin my blood. I had just gotten accepted to my residency program at UCLA- Harbor, my first choice. I thought, how many people get to live their dreams? My dream was to be a doctor and take care of people. That's my purpose. I love taking care of people. I live for taking care of people. I thought who could be luckier than me? I survived chemo, I survived mini-strokes, and blood clots in medical school. Even if I lived a short life, I lived a life of purpose in service to others, and so I was lucky.

So when the storms hit and the waters came, I thought, I can survive Hurricane Harvey. I will be okay. I always am. I'm always grateful in the moment for everything I have. I know no matter what storm comes through, I'll find a way through it. No matter how bad the storm gets, I will find the good, I will find the hope, I will choose to be lucky.

And yes it really is a choice. My grandmother told me the story of being released from the camps in Russia after the war. They were all unceremoniously dropped off at the train station to go back to Poland. After 2 years of forced labor, very little food, diseases, and despair, most of the people standing there didn't really resemble people anymore. My grandmother said they had no muscles on their arms and legs, and their bellies were swollen from starvation. They did not know if they would ever see their families again back in Poland, or whether any of them yet lived. My grandmother said she was standing there waiting for the train, and she heard someone in the train station playing music…and she started dancing. When she first told me that story, I asked her, how could you do that? How could you dance under those circumstances? She smiled at me and said, "because Brooksie, when you hear music, you dance." My grandmother only had a fourth grade education, and she is the wisest person I have ever met. She died last year at 99 years old, one of the last survivors of her generation and I miss her dearly. I still remember the sparkle in her eyes when she heard music, and up until she died, I played music for her and she would still tap her foot and smile.

All those years ago, when she stood in that train station, she could have been lost in thoughts about how awful she had been treated and felt depressed. She could have been worrying about what and who she will find in Poland and been anxious. She could have focused on her weary limbs and hungry belly. But instead, she found the music and she let joy enter her heart. If she could do that, then all of us can. We can face pain and illness and still choose to listen for the music. She taught me to choose.

So I refuse to choose suffering. You can be grateful and overwhelmed with gratitude, no matter how flooded you are or you can suffer even when the sun is shining. It's always your choice. You can make the choice to be grateful in this moment for who you are and everything you have, even if the storm is raging outside. I hope you do it. I feel grateful. I hope no matter where you are; whether it's pouring rain or whether the sun is shining, I hope you feel grateful too.

Chapter 12
Conquering Bad Habits To Master Success

You might have noticed that the Rapid Recovery protocol is more than just a nutrition plan. It's not just a diet. It's a learning experience. Once you start the Rapid Recovery plan, you will learn so much about yourself. Anything in your daily life at work or in your relationships that stops you in life will come up. You'll face your demons. Maybe you're a procrastinator who puts things off. You find that trying to drink a blender of smoothie is tough if you put it off to the end of the day. To be successful, you'll need to conquer your procrastination and change the bad habit. Maybe you're someone who has an addictive personality. You use food to help yourself feel better when you're struggling. If you're feeling achy or down, you eat. Now, you don't have that comfort food available. Conquering the cravings will be a big deal. If you're a pleaser, someone who feels like you're inconveniencing people, you may be tempted to go off the diet so you don't inconvenience people by standing out and saying you can't eat certain foods. Conquering that need to please everyone will be your struggle. Maybe you just feel unworthy of getting better. You feel you don't deserve this. You feel you don't deserve to get better. By conquering that doubt, you'll succeed with the protocol and beyond.

The best advice I can give you is: be aware. Notice when you're doing something that's hurting you or sabotaging you. Are you leaving the house without your water bottle? Are you eating the wrong foods because you're in a bad mood? What's pulling you away from the program? What is tempting you? Also ask yourself "why do I need to succeed in this?" Your success is important. You want to improve your life. Notice when you're being pulled off track, recognize it, and conquer the bad habit to succeed. I want you to succeed and I'm sure you want to succeed too.

Once you master your bad habits. Once you master not feeling worthy, or not wanting to be the odd one out in social situations, or not wanting to reach for a healthy snack instead of chocolate when you're in a bad mood, you will succeed on the diet and succeed in life. You'll succeed after six weeks and beyond. Healing takes place from the inside out.

Chapter 13
Self-Love Meditation

I wanted to share a meditation that can help you. If you're struggling with mindset, if you're feeling punished because you're dealing with illness, or you're feeling overweight or sluggish or unhappy with your body, this self-love meditation can really help. If it just feels like there's not much positive going on in your life and everything you want lies in another place, in another time, or you don't have what you need or what you want, try this meditation. If you are angry or resent your body for being sick, I hope it gives you some peace.

Happiness is always accessible to us. Even if you're sick, even if you're in pain, even if you don't look the way you want to look and your body's not working the way you want it to work, there's still happiness accessible to you. It comes from embracing what you have in the moment rather than feeling like the only way you can have happiness is if other things happen first, like being healthy. As long as you're stuck in that mindset, that you can only be happy when and if you get better, not now even while you are sick, success and happiness will always be one step away.

When I was on the high-dose steroids and taking chemotherapy and missing out on being a teenager because I was so sick, I was still happy because I focused on what I had, never what I lost. I had amazing parents and a family that loved me, a brain that worked really well, a good sense of humor, good friends. I saw the good in my life and I felt grateful for my body and my life, even when I was sick. My focus on gratitude helped me keep going while I was sick, and thrive at an even greater level once I was healthy.

Something I see holding people back in my Rapid Recovery Group is that they blame their body for their illness and pain. They see their body as their enemy. One of the revelations I guide them towards in the group is that their body is nor their enemy, but their best friend. Think about it: your body is fighting for you to stay alive in spite of everything you've ever done to it, eating toxic "foods", drinking alcohol, emotional, or physical abuse. It has survived infections and did not die. You and your body are on this earth together, and now is the time to stop abusing it; not just with the wrong foods, but with negativity, and anger and resentment. Healing is an act of self-love. Therefore, I want you to practice being loving to your body.

I want you to try this self-love meditation. I love it and I think you will too.

Close your eyes and relax, breathe deeply through your nose and out through your mouth. Feel the muscles in your body relax, starting with your toes, and all the way up your body to the top of your head.

When you are relaxed, I want you to start thanking yourself, one body part at a time. I want you to do it sincerely and with kindness in your heart.

Start with the tips of your toes. Say thank you to each part of your body for the things it does for you. Even if that part of your body doesn't work properly, even if it's in pain, even if it's paralyzed, I want you to thank that part of your body for what it's done for you or what it does for you.

For example, I'm going to start with my toes. Thank you to my toes that help me balance my feet so I don't fall over. Thank you to my feet that keep me balanced on the ground. They help me walk, they let me dance. If yours don't work for you anymore, perhaps you can remember a time you ran and thank your feet for that experience you had. Even if you're having trouble with a body party now, still find happiness and gratitude.

Move up through your legs; whether you think they're too fat or too skinny, whether they work right or whether they can't hold up your weight, thank your legs for what they've done for you. Then you move up into your pelvis and you thank yourself for the experiences you've had through your pelvis. Maybe you've delivered a baby, maybe you've had extraordinary sex. Maybe you're grateful you can eliminate toxins through your waste. Thank your pelvis for the function and joy it's given in your life.

Then you move into your stomach. Even if you're not happy with how a part of your body looks or how it works still take the time to thank it. My skin on my stomach is pretty stretchy after 2 kids, but I am so grateful I got to hold my babies in my belly and give them life. I am happy that my gut allows me to absorb nutrition from my diet. I can laugh when something tickles my belly. Search for positivity and gratitude for each part, and don't move on until you can give a truly sincere thank you to that part.

Remember to focus on each body part. Thank you to my lungs that still fill with air and allow me to breathe and allow me to speak and share my message and help others. Thank you to my heart that continues to beat every day. In spite of all of the medicines I put into my body, and all the illness I dealt with, my heart still continues to beat. It keeps me here and it keeps me on this earth.

Continue to move through your whole body. Your mouth that lets you share your heart. Say I love you to your nose that breathes for you even if it's crooked, and allows you to do the things you want to do. I say thank you to my brain for allowing me to have humor through the hardest parts of my life, to think of the words that people need to hear, to speak to my kids and tell them the wisdom I want them to know. Thank you to my ears, that can gain wisdom back into my body.

Move up through your body until you've completed all your thank yous. My hope is, during this meditation, you'll feel so grateful that happiness just pours out of you and pushes through your eyes as tears. These will be tears of happiness and joy, not pain or frustration.

I want you to go through step by step and, from your heart, thank each part of your body for what it's done for you and what it does for you. Feel that gratitude. If you can be grateful for a body that is sick, imagine what life will be like when you're healthy. Find your happiness here and today. Find your gratitude with what you have and who you are in this moment. Find happiness now. That happiness will only grow as you have more and more things to be grateful for as your body continues to heal and support you.

PART THREE
HABITS

"You are either in the habit of being sick, or you are in the habit of being healthy. If you want to change your health, you have to change your habits."
Dr. G

Chapter 14
All About Self Care

The reason self-care is an important part of the program is that we know from research and past client results, that high stress, high anxiety and depression increases your inflammation and slows down your healing.[14,15,16] It keeps you sick. Many people have difficulty getting better, not just because their nutrition isn't right, but because their lifestyle and their mood is keeping them sick. That is why self-care is a part of this healing protocol program. People who feel at peace and content and happy, get better much faster. Add healing foods like my green smoothies to your self-care and boom —take off to the finish line.

If you battle stress and anxiety every day, recovery is usually slower and there are more ups and downs. That doesn't mean you can't get better, it just means that in addition to great nutrition, you need amazing self-care to help you feel happy and relaxed and allow the nutrition to do its job. I want you to get good at maintaining a peaceful happy mood.

Self-care means time for relaxation and letting go of the stress of the day. It's the time when you breathe in deeply and sigh "ahhh" in relief. If you don't do that at least once a day, you are not taking good care of yourself. I want you to add self-care to your life. The first part of self-care is things you do on a daily basis to relax and let go of the stress of the day. It should be a daily ritual. There are so many things you can do to unwind and put the focus on you instead of everything else going on with life. Here are a few of my favorites:

*Meditation – I learned meditation as part of a training course to help people with chronic suicidality. People who are that depressed are often in their minds thinking about what they have lost or what they fear. I have found through my work with the chronically ill, that many of them are also depressed and scared and need help to be present in the moment. Meditation is one way to be in the moment in your body instead of in your thoughts. One way to do it is to focus on your breathing. Just noticing all the sensations that come with breathing: the feeling of air going into your nose, your chest expanding, the way the seat feels against your back as you inhale versus exhale, etc. If you have never meditated or have difficulty with the focus, that is normal. You can start with guided meditations that you just sit and listen to. There are many free guided meditations you can find online, or you use a meditation app or even go to a meditation class. Don't get mad at yourself if you're distracted during meditation at first. It takes time and practice.

*Coloring – Do you remember how calm you were as a kid just coloring away in your color book? You focused just on that and all the stress and worry melted away. You can do that again as an adult. Therapeutic coloring is wonderful. A study showed that coloring offers the same benefits as meditation![13] While the studies looked at coloring mandalas, and there are many Mandela coloring books available at art stores and online, I have found with my clients that there's no right or wrong color book. Color what makes you happy. Grab your kid's color book if you have nothing in particular in mind. Maybe you can color together. You're both relaxing!

*Being Out In Nature – There's a calmness in nature that is very beneficial to self-care. Sit under a tree, listen to the birds, or smell the flowers. Engage all of your senses while out in nature; focus on the sights, sounds and smells, and the feeling of the air on your skin. You can go to the ocean or a lake and immerse your senses there. The goal is to keep your focus outwards on the experience and not on thoughts.

*Take A Walk – walking helps calm us down, boosts creativity, and also is a great exercise. It also brings in the positive benefits of being out in nature. If you can't go outside for whatever reason, walking in place is just fine. There are some fabulous "virtual walk" videos online. You can walk to many places without ever leaving your home.

The next level of self-care is what I call bliss activities. Bliss means true happiness and joy. To experience bliss, you want to do more than just relax and unwind, you want to have fun or have top level nurturing. For bliss activities, find something that provides a huge lift to your spirit and makes you really happy. This is different for everyone. Think of yours. Is it travel? Is it going to see a live musical theater show? A day trip? How about a massage or a facial? How about seeing friends who always make you laugh until your cheeks hurt? You need something blissful to look forward to as often as possible. The excitement of planning your bliss and looking forward to it helps lift your mood. You've heard the expression "follow your bliss." Make sure to follow yours. It helps the healing process.

Thus, self-care consists of the activities you use to unwind and feel more peaceful and activities that give you bliss. If you can find peace and happiness even while being sick and symptomatic, then you don't have to wait to be healthy to be happy. If you've decided you won't be happy until you feel 100% healthy, then you will keep yourself from that goal. You need to find the peace and serenity and bliss here in this body even if it's got problems, because right now is all we have. The future hasn't happened yet. The past is over. Find happiness in this present day, in the present moment.

Chapter 15
Create A Sanctuary

I hope by now you are coming to understand that you don't need to just nourish your body in terms of the food that goes in, you need to nourish your spirit and your mental state. Stress, depression, and anxiety are all inflammatory.[14,15,16] Stress will battle against the anti-inflammatory food. That is why you need to incorporate self-care every day as I discussed in chapter 14. That is why self-care is on your list of things to fill out every day.

A space that helps you truly sink in and feel the stress leave your body. My sanctuary is my bathroom. I put a lot of love into this room. Every day I take an hour-long bath with Epsom or magnesium salts. I put essential oils in to make it smell great. I play beautiful music for myself. I relax. My work is intense, everyone I work with is in extreme pain. I love my work but it is definitely intense. I am also a mom and when I am not helping people get their health back I am taking care of my boys. I love my work and my family, and yet I still need time at the end of the day to just breathe and be peaceful by myself. My bath time is that time for me. When I sink into the hot water and smell the essential oils, my mind clears, my muscles relax and I feel drowsy and calm. Now, you don't need to make this your sanctuary, that is just my spot, but I want you to get creative with your favorite spot that is your special place to rest.

I have had many members of my rapid recovery programs who struggled with motivation, and much of the time it was because they did not do self-care. Their life was about work, family, taking care of their home, and eating on protocol, but they did not have a sanctuary or self-care ritual, and eventually they would fall back to using food for comfort because they didn't know a healthy way to soothe themselves. When I would encourage them to create their sanctuary and start doing self-care, they would give excuses like "it feels selfish", or "I am too busy." First of all, self-care isn't selfish, it's self-preservation! If you don't take care of yourself, mind, body, and spirit, you won't be able to keep taking care of anyone else. And for those that say they are too busy, I remind them that if you think you are too busy to take care of yourself, then eventually you will be too sick to be busy.

I had one client in my 6 Week rapid Recovery Group who resisted self-care for weeks. She told me that she was "not that kind of person", and was content just to work and care for her son and go to bed. I didn't buy it. Any time she had stress, like a fight with her husband, she would eat off plan. Why? Because she didn't have a way of soothing herself except through food. Therefore, not setting up a self-care plan was setting her up for self-sabotage anytime life got stressful, and eventually all of us face stress. She wanted to try taking long baths like me, but told me that every time she got into the tub, she felt her brain nagging her to get out and go be productive and she would get out of the tub. One day she decided to give in to my advice and stay in the tub. She said the nagging voice persisted for 10 minutes, and then suddenly it stopped and she felt herself relax and sink into the water. The next thing she knew, she was sobbing in the tub. She told me that she realized at that moment that it was the very first time she had ever done something just to allow herself to feel good. From that moment on she was a convert, and religiously took her long baths every night. She felt happier, was able to easily commit to her nutrition plan without any more incidents of eating off plan, and she completely eliminated lupus from her life. She now has normal laboratory tests, and has 2 healthy kids.

In addition to baths, clients in my Rapid Recovery Group have created a special spot with a soft comfortable chair, pictures of their favorite memories and scented candles, or some will have a spot in their backyard where they love to sit under a tree and listen to birds chirping as they have their smoothie. Another set up an easel to start painting again, a pleasure she had given up long ago that brought her so much happiness and peace. Your sacred space is your designated space to let of your stress and worries and be present in the moment.

Assignment:

Your assignment is to create your sanctuary. It can be a simple desk, it can be a wall on a room, it can be a corner, or it can be a walk-in closet. The key is you need a space that's yours to restore your peace.

What I encourage you to do is use your 5 senses to create your sanctuary. The five senses are sight, hearing, touch, smell, and taste. When you focus on your senses, it connects you to your body. You can't be in your head if you're in your body. Also, your body is always in the present, not in the past or the future, which means that when you use your 5 senses you are practicing mindfulness meditation. For example, here is how I use my 5 senses in my bathtub:

1. Sight: I dim the lights and use candles and I have a beautiful painting hanging in front of my tub to look at.
2. Sound: I brought in a speaker to listen to spa music or classical music.
3. Touch: I feel the hot water softened by the bath salts against my skin and the humidity against my face.
4. Smell: scented bath salts or essential oils.
5. Taste: I will have a mug of peppermint tea to sip on while I soak.

When people finally and truly start scheduling in time just for themselves to feel good, they feel more motivated to eat the right foods, as well as more energetic to do all the other things they need to in their lives. Then the nutrition plan becomes simple, because food is for fuel and disease reversal, not an emotional crutch.

Chapter 16
Good Sleep Hygiene

Sleep is essential for healing and good health. Sleep is the primary time in your day your body works on repairing itself. Sleep disruption is associated with increased activity of the sympathetic nervous system, and your adrenal glands. It also causes metabolic effects like weight gain and heart disease, and has been shown to be proinflammatory.[17,18] In otherwise healthy adults, short-term consequences of sleep disruption include increased stress, increased pain in their bodies, increased emotional distress and mood disorders, and problems with thinking and memory.[17,19] I have observed the negative effects of sleep deprivation many times in my 6 Week Rapid Recovery Group. The most common symptom of sleep deprivation is lack of energy and brain fog. I had one group member who kept complaining that she didn't feel the high energy that the other group members were feeling on the nutrition plan, but she was only getting 3 to 6 hours of sleep a night! You can't expect to have energy if you are sleep deprived! Another person was eating according to plan but not getting the same rapid reduction in her symptoms as fellow group members and she was very upset about it. She also would get 3 to 4 hours of sleep a night. She had a long history of insomnia and struggled in this area. We worked on attacking this issue in multiple areas: first making peace that she would go slower but still be improving her health because in spite of her poor sleep, she was still nourishing her body and doing self-care which decreases inflammation. The poor sleep was just going to slow down her results until she got a handle on it. The second thing we did was encourage naps – sleep when you can, especially during the healing process. While a continuous night of sleep is optimal, you need to sleep when you can and do your best to rest when your body is willing to. The third thing we worked on is something called sleep hygiene.

Sleep hygiene is simply a term that refers to sleep hygiene in a variety of different practices and habits that are necessary to have good nighttime sleep quality. The most important component of good sleep hygiene is having a routine at bedtime that helps signal to your brain it's time to shut down. Our brains like habit. They like routine. Now that also works for sleep. You want a ritual in place where your brain knows it's time for sleep. When you create your sleep ritual, make sure it is calming and you should stick to it religiously. I had a group member who was exhausted because she was up until 2:00am cleaning her floors. I told her that the dirt on the floor won't change her health, but prioritizing clean floors over sleep will rob her of her recovery. I had her agree to a bed time that was written in stone, dirty house or not, and when she did, her energy and mood came up quickly.

What does a sleep routine look like? That depends on you. Your ideal bedtime is usually the time of night when you notice yourself starting to get tired. Many people push through the first signs of sleepiness to other tasks, and then the sweet spot for sleep passes and they start to become more awake again. Notice when you feel tired and aim for that to be your bedtime, even if it's earlier than you would normally choose for yourself. You need to prioritize your sleep while you are trying to recover your health. When you are healthy your sleep needs will naturally decrease.

If your ideal bedtime is 10:00pm, then you can start your routine at 8:30pm: you can have a glass of chamomile tea while reading a fun book (nothing too serious or engaging that will keep you up late), or have a long shower, or stretch and listen to relaxing music. Then maybe at 9:30pm be in your pajamas and listen to a guided meditation. At 10:00pm turn off the lights and let go of your day. That is just one example, you can create your own routine, just make sure it is 1) scheduled 2) consistent, 3) calming and relaxing 4) no electronics at least 2 hours before you go to sleep.

Another part of sleep hygiene, and a big problem for many, is when the bed and the bedroom is being used for too many things: sleep, reading, watching TV, studying, etc. What happens when the bedroom is used for too many non-sleep related activities? Your brain gets confused over what the bedroom is for. Your brain makes connections between your rituals and how you feel. For example, if you have a ritual of eating while you watch TV, then often as soon as you sit down on the couch to watch TV, you feel hungry. Are you actually hungry? Well, not necessarily but your brain has now made an association that TV watching means eating time. It's why when you go to a restaurant, even if you're not hungry, when you sit at the table suddenly you are. Your brain has associated those things together.

One of the best things you can do if you have trouble sleeping is make sure your bedroom, and specifically your bed, is only a place for sleep (and sex). If you're working in bed, reading in bed, watching TV in bed, snacking in bed, your brain will not know why it's there. When you get into bed, your brain is not going to know if it needs to be alert, relaxed, or sleepy.

You want it to be clear for your mind that sleep is the only reason you are in bed. If you want to read before bed, have a chair near your bed for reading. Move into bed when you're feeling sleepy. While you're lying in bed, it's okay to play a guided sleep meditation. That helps your mind relax and focus on the voice of the meditation leading you into relaxation rather than being alert and active listening to a TV show or movie before bed. Make sure your bedroom is a place to rest.

Remember, here are the three steps to better sleep hygiene:

1. Make yourself sleep rituals or a sleep schedule.
2. Start your sleep schedule at the same time every night.
3. Make sure your bedroom is a place for sleep and sex – nothing else.

I hope that helps you get started with a long-lasting routine that will help you optimize your sleep which also helps you optimize your healing and your health.

Chapter 17
Counting Your Celebrations

After many years of coaching people through the disease-reversal programs, I have discovered that celebrating is an important habit for success with healing – and anything in life that you are trying to do.

Celebration is big. My husband did a study once with people trying to lose weight. He asked them to jot down everything they did wrong in the past five days about their exercise and nutrition. They wrote it down while he timed them. Then he said, "now I want you to write five things you did right over the past five days." He timed them again. What he found was that the people who could write down what they did right and wrong in the same time frame were the ones with the best weight loss results. There were other folks who took only 5 minutes to write down a long list of everything they were doing wrong, yet it took them 15 or even 30 minutes to come up with only 5 things they did right. Those people had very slow to no results. Why would that be? Because people who are good at finding faults with themselves and struggle to think about things they do right, are in the habit of criticizing themselves but not in the habit of celebrating themselves. When you feel constantly criticized, like you can't do anything right, do you feel more motivated or less motivated? Most people feel depressed, unmotivated, and like a failure, and people who feel like that tend to put in low effort or quit. They set themselves up for failure. When people can quickly come up with things they need to work on and also recognize the things they are doing right, they feel motivated by the successes and can plan to do better on the things they are doing wrong. We need to celebrate what is going right to have the energy to fix the things we still need to work on.

Think of it like this: Whatever you did wrong is information, and you can use this information to make decisions that increase the right things and decrease the wrong things. Whatever you did right is cause for celebration.

Think about how celebrations affect your motivation to do things. Here's a quick example: kindergarten graduation. Why do we have a graduation party for kindergarteners when they've got twelve more grades to do? Because the excitement of the celebration keeps them motivated to go back and do more school. Imagine those little kids finishing their first year of school and all we said was, "no big deal, there's 12 more years to go", rather than clapping and hugging them and telling them how proud we are. Do you think they would want to keep learning? Not at all. Why work hard for no reward, emotional or otherwise?

We want to celebrate every little victory so we keep going. If you're focused on what you did wrong, if you feel like every day is a failure, why would you want to do that again? Why work so hard? I want you to write something down in celebrations every day. Not something sarcastic like "I didn't hate the kale smoothie", but something genuine. Even if it's "I did another day on this diet and this is the hardest thing I ever did and I am proud of myself", be proud of yourself for trying. Be proud of yourself for continuing. Every day you get this right, be proud of yourself. Every day you just did better than you did the day before, be proud of yourself for that. Every day you wake up and get out of bed, be proud of yourself for that. The full healing protocol is difficult but it's worth it. If you let yourself celebrate every little victory, you will be more motivated to keep working hard at it until you get the hang of it.

In my Rapid Recovery programs, my clients have a daily workbook to share with me, that notes their foods, their sleep, their moods, their pain, and also has a space for celebrations. Sometimes I will have participants write "none" or "I woke up today" under the success portion of their daily workbook, something negative or sarcastic that shows they are only seeing their pain and their problems. Those people usually struggle with the program, eating off plan, noting more depression and anxiety, and do not follow through on the support I offer them. I work with them on taking their focus completely off the struggles (they are already very aware of them because they think about them all day), and instead work on writing down 5 things going well every day. I choose 5 because you really need to sit and think to come up with 5 things. I encourage them to understand that we always find what we are looking for; so, if we are used to looking for pain and failure, that is all we see. When we start truly searching for beauty, love and success, we will notice it all around us. As they get better at celebrating, their moods improve and their dedication too.

Another important part of celebrating is finding something to be happy about every single day. If you can find one thing to give you joy that day, even if it's small, celebrate that. If you can find one thing that makes you happy every day, that means your happiness does not depend on everything being perfect in your life or in your health. That means you can be happy even if you're sick. You can enjoy your life even if you don't have your health. If you can do that, things will only get better and better. If you can be happy now—if you can find joy now—then healing is just a bonus. That's what I want for you. I was sick for many years but it never took my joy away. I focused on my strengths and gratitude every day, and I focused on fun and purpose. That habit of joy and celebration kept me happy even while I was sick, and ultimately made it easy for my body to heal once I added the nutrition it had been starving for, for so long. The combination of low stress, gratitude and joy, and the right nutrition is the path to rapid recovery of your health and also success at everything else you put your mind to. Remember, when you're depressed, when you're anxious, when you're down, your inflammation levels go up. If you find your peace and joy and something to make you happy in each day, then you can enjoy your life even as you heal, and you will heal faster.

Assignment:

Start a Success Journal. At the end of every day, write down at least 5 things that you did well or that made you happy that day. I want you to write your celebrations – the good in your life and your success with healing process – every day.

PART FOUR
ISSUES & SELF-SABOTAGE

Chapter 18
Being Good at Healing Makes You Good At Life

For healing, it's not just about having the right information about what to eat. Healing is about the actions you take on the information; what you do that holds you back or stops you, and what you do that gets you results. I assess people's motivation by how they talk about obstacles. For example, if someone has an event coming up where there is unhealthy foods, sometimes they will tell me, "oh you know what? Maybe I'll start Monday. I'm going to be at a party, so I won't be able to eat right on Sunday," or they'll say "oh well you know there's a barbeque so that night I'm going to eat badly, but then I'll eat better in other days." In all of these cases, the people are looking for reasons not to do the program. They are looking for reasons to quit, slow down, or fail. They're looking for a reason to sabotage themselves.

Someone who is motivated to succeed will ask these kind of questions instead:

- "How can I eat healthy at the party on Sunday night?"
- "Can you give me advice on how to nourish myself at the BBQ?"
- "Can you tell me how to talk to people at the party who might question or make fun of my food choices?"

Those questions show me the person is searching for ways to succeed at recovering their health. They see the potential obstacles but are looking for ways around them, rather than seeing them seeing them as a reason to quit. Someone who wants to win sees potential obstacles and asks "What do I need to do to make sure I stay healthy?" That's the mindset of someone who will heal their body. They're not looking for a reason to fail. They're looking for a reason to succeed. They are chasing their health like a dog chasing an ambulance. Full speed ahead. Nothing will stop them. Someone who makes excuses is still looking for reasons to fail and not looking for reasons to succeed. Know of your mindset. Do you want to fail or succeed? Do your actions support what you really want?

Another downfall to healing is that a lot of people don't prioritize themselves. I see this predominantly in women, but sometimes in men as well. I call it Mother Martyr Syndrome. Ladies, especially moms, are often great at putting everyone else first. They will wake up and give their kids breakfast and make sure their husband is taken care of. They'll go to work and work hard at their jobs. They'll come home and make dinner and clean the house and basically work until the moment they pass out at night. Then they say they didn't have time for their smoothie, their self-care, or their workout. If you're not prioritizing yourself, you will be sick. If you're not sick now, you will get sick. We cannot run on adrenaline and caffeine alone. If you are the one taking care of other people, you've got to have the best self-care. If you don't, you're sabotaging your success. Remember, if you think you are too busy to take care of yourself, you will eventually be too sick to be busy.

Reversing your disease will not be convenient and will not be easy, but it is worth it. Your health is everything, you need to treat it the way. I am a queen of self-care. I prioritize myself. I make sure I get great sleep. I make sure I'm drinking my green smoothies and water every single day. I make sure I have my time for meditation. I make time for my long baths. At the time of this publication, I will be lupus-free for 14 years and counting. I don't want to just be lupus free, I want to have extraordinary health, and I do. I want you to have extraordinary health too. If you are not prioritizing your health, that is a problem. It will catch up to you. You won't heal and get healthy if you don't make yourself a priority. And Moms: Take great care of yourself so you can enjoy being a mom. Don't teach your kids how to not prioritize their health. Teach your kids how to take care of themselves by showing them a supreme example of how to do it. If you have think of taking care of yourself as something you do for them, then do it. Just make sure you think of your health first, or you won't have the ability to take care of anyone else.

One of my clients in my Rapid Recovery Group was having difficulty staying with the nutrition plan because she was a mom and a grandmother and a wife, and her kids, grandkids, and her husband were her entire focus. Genie is one of the case studies in the next section. She made their food, she homeschooled her grandkids, she did everything for them, and developed lupus along the way. When I met her, she was exhausted, in pain, and depressed. She had tried to do the protocol on her own but always gave up on herself. She finally decided to join the 6 Week Rapid Recovery Group so I could give her daily help and support to overcome the barriers and finally get her health back. I discovered that she was a Mom Martyr! She was willing to literally kill herself to support her family, but didn't see the value of taking care of herself.

When I started asking her to take care of herself with self-care, she kept giving me reasons why she was too busy to do it. I stuck with her and she decided that an extended soak in a hot bath would be very nice at the end of a long day of taking care of her grandkids. She first needed to realize that what she was doing was unsustainable. She was getting sicker and sicker, so how was she going to take care of anyone else if she was dying herself? I gave her permission to tell her family she was having private time and to lock her door. Her husband could handle the kids for a while if he needed to. She felt enormous relief and peace to have even 30 minutes to rest quietly in her tub without worrying about anyone or anything else. She experienced a dramatic emotional shift when finally decided to stop living only for others and start taking care of herself. She found that her energy was better, her mood was better, and she no longer felt the stress she normally did. She said that the things that caused her stress didn't change; she just didn't experience it the same way anymore. Her cravings for comfort foods like cookies and soda went away. She put herself first, felt cared for by herself, and started healing. By the end of the 6 weeks, she had energy, little to no pain, and she reversed her anti-phospholipid antibodies so she no longer had to worry about having a stroke.

Anything you're doing that's hurting you out there in the world will show up when you're trying to heal yourself. If you are someone who puts yourself last in your relationships, that habit will be an obstacle to your healing. If you're someone who looks for excuses or sabotages yourself because you have issues around your own worthiness or your belief in yourself, it will show up when you're trying to heal. There are many ways your mind will try to stop you. Some common behaviors that I see often in my rapid recovery program are procrastinating, people-pleasing, and addictive behavior.

Procrastinating - You're used to putting things off until the last minute, so you start eating too late in the day and then find yourself trying to drink 50 ounces of smoothie at 8pm. Then you're up all night using the bathroom. You're suffering because of the procrastination.

Solution: You need to schedule your food preparation and eating times. Planning beats procrastinating.

People-Pleasing– You're uncomfortable putting somebody out or feeling like you're inconveniencing someone. It may tempt you to go off the diet because you don't want that person to feel bad or you hate standing out.

Solution: Eating raw vegetables and not eating meat or cheese is going to seem odd to others who are still immersed in their own food addictions and traditions. You need to make peace with that. It is not your job to make other people happy or comfortable, how people feel is entirely up to them and their own inner work, not up to you. Even if you kill yourself trying to please others, you won't have made them happy, but just caused your own demise. You don't owe anyone an explanation or need to eat something that you know is bad for you, even if someone made it for you. You can be kind and grateful and still stick with what is right for you. No one else will do this for you, you have to decide you are worth it.

Addictive Eating – You use food as an emotional crutch, both as a reward for a job well done and for comfort when you're feeling down. If you use food to bring you comfort and now you don't have those foods available anymore, you will have a tough time with cravings.

Solution: Use relationships and activities to create happiness, not food (See Chapter 24).

What I find sometimes in this program is maybe there's a part of you that's been really hurt, that feels unworthy of all of the great things you will receive and that part of you sabotages you. Notice when you're doing something that's hurting you or sabotaging you. Are you leaving the house without your water bottle? Are you eating the wrong foods because you're in a bad mood or is it because you're in a social situation? What's coming up for you that pulls you away from the program? What is it that's tempting you? When you're aware of this, write it down. Ask yourself what the triggers are for you to take that action. Then follow that up with why you need to succeed at this?

Your success is so important. You want to improve your life. Any time you're getting pulled away from that, I just want you to notice it. I want you to write it down. When you can master your cravings, when you can master how to handle a social situation where you feel you're the weird one out or you might inconvenience people, when you can master how to handle a bad mood without going for chocolate, when you can master your diet in the face of all the real world drama that pulls you off your game, then you will not only master your diet, you will be a master at life. You will be in control of your health and your happiness.

When you truly start to put yourself first, nurture your spirit and nourish your body, that is when healing happens. And that is why being good at healing, makes you good at life. Your self-esteem will improve, your relationships will improve, you'll perform better at work. Take care of yourself. Stop making excuses. Look for how you will get it done instead of why you can't.

When you do that, not only will you heal your body, but you will have gotten really good at living your best life.

Chapter 19
Identifying and Eliminating Unsupportive Thoughts

The main cause of your successes and failures is not what is happening around you, it is the thoughts and beliefs you have about the things happening around you. How you interpret what's happening to you will determine how you feel and what you do. People who self-sabotage give up or do things that slow themselves down from obtaining their goals, tend to have what I call negative mental habits. Mental habits are the way you normally think about things. Are your thoughts generally optimistic? Then you have positive mental habits like looking at the bright side, minimizing negative events and focusing on gratitude. If you find you are more accustomed to finding faults, worrying about what can go wrong, or minimizing the good things in your life, you have some negative mental habits.

If we have mental habits that are causing more suffering, we'll have less happiness. Even if you are eating perfectly according to the protocol, your mental habits may cause more suffering even as your body is trying to eliminate inflammation and recover from disease. Because this is a key source of emotional distress and self-sabotage, I spend time in my 6 Week Rapid Recovery Group teaching the members about these mental habits and helping them identify the ones they have used or still use to stop themselves. Here are some common ones I have come across in my clients. If any of these pertain to you, I want you to write them down. Own it. Say "that's me." Think about how those habits caused you undue suffering.

SHOULD-ING – This mental habit causes people a lot of pain and anxiety. People with this habit believe there is a way that things should be, or things that they should be able to do or have. People often should on others, "he should know better", or "they should know what I really mean/want (even if I didn't explicitly say it)". There is no one way that things are supposed to be, there is only the way that it is. The power we have, is to change the way things are. Lamenting about the way we think it should be creates sadness, anxiety, and inertia. Do you find yourself stuck in shoulds? Ever think, "I should be healthy, I eat better than my friends"? I hear that one a lot. Or "I eat mostly on plan, I should feel better." How about, "If I am getting better, I shouldn't be so tired." That one implies that you would know what it feels like to heal from a disease when you have never done it before, which gives you reason to quit before you experience the changes you seek. When you're in the land of should, there's a lot of suffering. You're not accepting what your life is. When I had lupus, my mother didn't let me sink into sadness about my life being different than others, she instead had me focus on my purpose and my gifts. I learned the best path forward was not thinking about what my life should be like as a 16 year old girl, but rather, "what do I need to do to keep living and create the best life possible for myself?" When you are stuck in "should", you create pain and suffering while also shutting your creativity for finding answers. If you catch yourself thinking that way, write it down and think about how it hurts your life. Then focus on the present, on the way things are, and how you plan to improve the things that you have the power to change.

FORTUNE TELLING – This mental habit is one that I frequently see in my clients who have a history of self-sabotage and giving up. This is that habit of believing that if you think about something long enough, you can predict what will happen. If I eat too much fat, I will ruin my thyroid. If I don't eat fruit, I will have less energy. If I stay up too late, my family will be disappointed in me. In a recent group, my client discovered that she sabotages herself by telling herself "if Dr. G wants me to be raw forever, I can't do that, it'll be too hard". She made up a future that is not accurate (I never said she has to stay raw and she didn't ask), and then decided based on the imaginary future she came up with, that she couldn't do the program. She effectively stopped herself before she started, all in her own mind. If you're stuck in fortune telling, you're not in reality. You're causing suffering for yourself in an imaginary world that doesn't exist in the here and now. The things you are predicting will likely never happen, but you still suffer as if they do. You're stuck in a negative place because you're trying to predict what will happen before it happens, and unless you are an incredible psychic, you probably are terrible at it like everyone else. Fortune telling is a mental habit that takes you out of the game and stops you before you even truly try. If this is you, say that's me. Own it. Think about how it has robbed you of your happiness. Catch yourself doing it and stop yourself. None of us know what will happen. If something bad happens, we'll fix it. If you're sitting there waiting to figure out what will happen ahead of time, you will always be standing still. You will never get closer to your dream or your happiness.

DISQUALIFYING THE POSITIVE – This is a common habit for people with depression and with negative beliefs about their own self-worth. When you disqualify the positive, you ignore the positive things that are happening and only focus on the negative ones. I had a client who did 4 Weeks of Rapid Recovery with me, who came to me with terrible hip pain. This pain stopped her from walking and she was stuck in bed. It took 28 days for that particular pain to go away, and for 27 of those 28 days, she told me the protocol wasn't working. Now while that pain was still there, she experienced an abundance of other benefits: her swelling was gone, the arthritis in her hands was gone, her energy was better, her skin was glowing. All of these positive things were happening but she looked only at the negative. She disqualified every positive thing that happened and only focused on the one negative. She then used that negative to decide nothing good was happening in spite of all of the evidence to the contrary. She wanted to keep the negative narrative in her head. She created misery and despair for herself by disqualifying the positive, when she could have been experiencing excitement and hope by looking at all of the positives. Imagine if instead, during the weeks leading up to day 28, she had been celebrating her wins and counting all the new benefits and positive changes? Then even as she waited for a change in her hip pain, she could have been happy and excited. People always find what they are looking for: if you are looking for what's wrong, you will always find it, and if you are looking for what's right, you will always find it. If you find this one is a habit of yours, write it down, reflect on the pain it has caused you, and start a success journal for yourself where you write down 5 things every day that are going well! Don't ignore those positives any longer!

ALL OR NOTHING THINKING – If you have this mental habit, you tend to either think the best or worst of everything and everyone. There's no in between. Someone is amazing or they are a demon. A program is the best thing ever or a total nightmare. The truth is, no person or thing is ever all good or all bad, and when you allow yourself to think so, you will have a tendency to walk away from people or programs when you see what you perceive to be a flaw or a negative, because if that happens, you will decide he/she/it is bad and quit. I see this happen in my Rapid Recovery programs sometimes. As part of the program I need to give people daily feedback and sometimes really confront them with the thoughts or behaviors that I observe are keeping them sick. It is essential to their recovery that I do that, but this is tricky ground because if the person has had traumatic or unhealthy relationships in the past, this can feel like criticism and make them angry. Because I am aware of this issue, I always ask permission to confront them when we start the program, to prepare them for it, and I am always as gentle as I can be, but sometimes people still get upset. Now I encourage open communication and expression, and we are almost always able to work through the feelings together and often have incredible breakthroughs because of this emotional work. However, if someone has all or nothing thinking, and gets angry at my feedback, there is a chance he or she can decide I am not actually a good person and quit. The reality is, good and nice people sometimes say things that can hurt, but it doesn't mean they aren't good. Sometimes it is painful to realize certain things about your behavior, thoughts or motivation, and yet it takes a kind helping person to point it out to you and help you overcome it. Sometimes someone loving and supportive can accidentally trigger you and cause you pain.

There is one client recently who did the 6 Week Rapid Recovery Group who joined the group to beat autoimmune disease. She couldn't believe how much she got out of the program: she was able to get a hold of a lifelong eating disorder with our help and process devastating childhood traumas through our forgiveness work and told us she had found peace that a lifetime of therapy never gave her. She thought my husband and I were angels in her life and happily decided to stay for another 6 weeks to keep up the support to get her even healthier. During one live meeting, someone asked my husband about his favorite restaurants in Houston and he talked about a vegan buffet he likes that has unhealthy vegan foods. He also said that this is not a place for the rapid recovery phase but for when you are healthy and want to have occasional recreational eating. This client got very triggered by his excitement over recreational eating, although she didn't mention it during the meeting. She eventually brought it up in group that she felt triggered and hurt by his behavior because she has an eating disorder and would not be able to balance recreational and nutritional eating and stopped posting for the rest of the group. She negated all of the good he had brought to her life over the previous months and instead only saw a man who triggered negative emotions, and she walked away. Because of that all-or-nothing thinking, she stopped herself from continuing to get help and support that had changed her life up until that point, help that could have brought so much more healing. We apologized for triggering her, and offered to help her process her feelings and keep going, but regretfully she didn't return.

The opposite can also be true: people with all or nothing thinking can sometimes continue unhealthy relationships because a person was initially kind and they decided he was "good" and then ignored evidence to the contrary and stay in an abusive relationship because they are unable to see the nuances, that there are positives and negatives to every person. Our triggers come from our personal pains and traumas, and kind well-meaning people can sometimes trigger you because they didn't know that pain was there, like stepping on a hidden landmine. It is important to become aware of our triggers, communicate to others what they are, and also remember that the triggers exist because of old wounds, so that you don't take out your pain and anguish on new people who accidentally trigger you. This is very difficult work that you want to engage a therapist to help you with. If you want to overcome the mental habit of all or nothing thinking, then one activity that can help is to work on finding balance between positives and negatives. For example, if you are unsure about a relationship, trying making a pros and cons list about that person's behavior and decide whether you want him or her in your life based on the pros vs. cons, instead of passing judgment on a person being all "good" or "bad". Everyone, including yourself, has positive and negative qualities, and you need to give everyone space for mistakes, especially yourself. If someone is a consistently hurtful presence in your life, let them go. If someone is helpful and loving but sometimes accidentally triggers you, talk with them about your triggers and give them the chance to be considerate of your sensitivities as your work on them in your own psychotherapy.

I hope this list helps you minimize your suffering and move forward with having the most abundant, happy life. If you find that you have more than one of these mental habits and also suffer from anxiety or depression, I encourage you to explore cognitive behavioral psychotherapy approaches that help you learn how to rewire your thinking to support more happiness and health. You deserve the best healing and health possible.

Chapter 20
How To Interpret A Bad Day

Bad days happen. It's normal. We all have bad days. Maybe you got stressed out and made a choice that hurt your body, or the stress itself created inflammation and you experienced more pain. Maybe you got a stomach virus. and couldn't eat your healing foods for a few days. Maybe you had too little sleep last night and your pain feels worse today. All types of stressors affects our bodies, especially our energy, pain, and inflammation levels. Also, during early rapid recovery, people often have a few days of no pain or great energy, and then experience a day of low energy or a resurgence of symptoms over the normal course of reversing their disease. When people see those symptoms as normal ups and downs, and just sleep more and do more self-care on bad days without attaching negative thoughts or emotions to it, they recover quickly and usually feel better than ever within a day or two. However, when people have a bad day and then attach a negative meaning to those symptoms, they create more stress, and thereby more inflammation in addition to creating unnecessary emotional upset.

Just because you have a bad day where you have more pain or less energy doesn't mean you're not doing better. It just means you have more symptoms that day. One example I see a lot in my 6 Week Rapid Recovery Group is that someone will have a high energy day and use that energy to do many things they normally don't feel up to, like working out or running errands. Then the next day they feel tired and don't want to get out of bed. The low energy does not mean they are not getting better. They had a low energy day because they did more than they're used to the day before. They spent more energy than they are used to and their body needs to recover. The protocol is still working. The fact that the high energy day happened at all is evidence of recovery. If you don't stress out and continue taking great care of yourself, soon you'll have constant energy instead of highs and lows.

While some people in recovery feel better each day moving in a linear way towards being pain free, some people find their pain levels (or other symptoms) vacillate up and down like a stock ticker as they move towards becoming symptom free. Whereas they used to be in constant pain, their pain will become variable with ups and downs. There will be high pain days followed by low to no pain days, and then higher pain again and low to no pain again, etc., rather than it hurting less and less each day. Symptoms come and go, energy comes and goes. Pain comes and goes, rashes or swelling comes and goes. Now this is a big improvement from the symptoms being there all the time, and a good sign of disease reversal, however don't let your mood go up and down with the symptoms; happy on days with low to no symptoms, depressed and hopeless on days with more symptoms. Use the skills like self-care and positive self-talk that I taught you in previous chapters to keep your mood peaceful, positive and steady even while your symptoms fluctuate, to minimize stress and emotional distress.

Also, make sure you focus on the good and the positive. If you had a good day yesterday, remind yourself that that is a great indicator that you are indeed getting healthier, and that a bad day just means you need more rest or self-care. Remember how you interpret things affects your mood which affects your inflammation. If you go "Man that hip pain is not better yet. I'm a failure. It will never work." Boom! You get inflammation going up in your bloodstream from all that negative stress and depression. How you interpret things affects how you will heal. Just because you still have some problems left doesn't mean you're not getting better. If you're not where you want to be yet, it's not because the things you're doing will not get you there.

Three things to remember about self-sabotage and bad days are:

1. Remind yourself that a bad day does not mean the protocol is not working or that you cannot get your health back. Instead, notice what your symptoms are: evaluate a) is there an explanation for more inflammation today, like poor sleep, more stress, eating off plan, or eating a new food that might be causing a sensitivity? Then, b) plan to solve any issues you come up with and then nourish your body on protocol and nourish your spirit with self-care and rest.
2. Focus on what is better, not on what is wrong or still bothering you. Maybe your hip still hurts, but your energy is better so celebrate that.
3. Focus on the positives in your life, and don't use fortune-telling, or discounting the positives to create a negative narrative for yourself. Mindset and self-talk is vital to your recovery. By focusing on the good, you'll find motivation to keep doing more and, most importantly, to keep getting better.

What gives you the energy and the drive to move forward? Focus on what's going well. Remember how you interpret and judge what's going right or wrong will affect your mood and your recovery. Don't judge how well you're doing. Focus on self-care and what is in your power to do. I want you to take amazing care of yourself on a tough day. I want you to love yourself. I want you to be proud of yourself. One bad day will not ruin your healing journey, it's just a part of the journey.

Chapter 21
How To Have Pain Without Suffering

As you may have surmised from the previous chapter, the biggest suffering we have is often not because of the pain we're going through, but because the meaning we give to the pain. One example of this is having a bad day, like I discussed in the last chapter. For example, someone on the protocol is doing great. Her energy is amazing, her pain is gone, everything is working. Then she has a bad day. She has a stomachache and just feels terrible. What is true in that moment is she's having stomach pains. That is absolutely what's happening. That is observing what it is, noticing the symptoms without diagnosing it, giving it meaning, or predicting anything based on it. Now there doesn't have to be suffering just because there's pain. Suffering happens when you make the pain mean something negative. If the pain means "everybody has a bad day let me just do what I need to do and tomorrow will be better," then you can accept the pain without suffering and focus on problem solving the source of the pain and self-care. That's the mindset you want. But if you create a negative meaning around the pain, like "I will never be healthy", there will be suffering. Suffering is the emotional distress caused by the negative thinking about the symptoms. It's the depression. It's the hopelessness. That's where suffering comes from. The meaning we give things causes our suffering, not the pain itself.

Sometimes I see people in my 6 Week Rapid Recovery group cause themselves suffering when they see others doing well. People get better at different rates and different days in the group, depending on their symptoms, their illness, their dedication to the nutrition plan and the self-care, their sleep, etc. I encourage members to celebrate with the group every time they feel better, so they can practice celebrating, and to inspire others who are still struggling that they too will get better as long as they keep going. However, I have had members who were in the habit of creating suffering for themselves with negative assumptions and mental habits. Those members will see group members doing well, and instead of thinking, "Wow if they can heal and they can feel great then so can I", they will get depressed reading about another's member's success and comment, "they get to feel good and I don't. I'll never heal. I'm not like them. This isn't for me." Everyone witnessed the same event, but the interpretation they give it either creates excitement or suffering. Do you see the difference? There's suffering with the negative meaning. Be very careful in the meaning you give things.

If you experience a bad day, negative symptoms, or if you're still in pain and still struggling to recover, just notice it like a reporter taking down the news. Tell yourself "Oh, this is happening today. I have pain in my legs today. My energy is low today." Don't put meaning on it. Just note that it's there and then go into problem solving mode, 1) is there a trigger I can identify so I can try to avoid it in the future, and 2) what can I do to feel better today? Don't add any meaning or emotion to it. If you avoid put negative meaning and emotions on symptoms, you can still feel happy even while you have pain, and that is how you have pain without suffering.

Chapter 22
Meditation To Find Limiting Beliefs

If you find you are in the habit of sabotaging yourself, you might have some negative or limiting beliefs about yourself, health, healing, or others that are holding you back from going all out in your recovery. This is a meditation I created for my 6 Week Rapid Recover group to help members identify their limiting beliefs and commit themselves fully to their recovery. This meditation has been eye-opening and revelatory for many members.

You can either read this chapter and then do the exercise on your own, you can record yourself reading it and then play it for yourself with your eyes closed or you can have a friend read it to you while you relax and dive into the experience.

Make sure you've got a quiet place to yourself. Get comfortable, you can lie down or sit. If you're sitting, you can stretch your feet out in front of you or plant your feet on the ground, don't cross your legs. Have your hands resting on your lap with your palms facing up. If you're lying down, make sure you're relaxed with your eyes closed. Wherever you are, make sure you're in a quiet room where you feel safe and calm. Take some deep breaths. Breathe in through your nose, hold it for two beats, then release it through your mouth for four counts. Breathe in (one, two). Breathe out (one, two, three, four). Focus on the sensation of your breath and relaxing, sinking into your chair or bed, and keep doing that until you feel your body relax.

Next, you will focus on relaxing each part of your body. Start with your feet. Feel all the muscles of your feet and toes relax, let go of tension and let them go limp. Move up to your legs. Your calves. Release the tension and stress, let go. Keep breathing. With each exhale, let go more deeply. Let your body sink further and further into relaxation. Breathe in. Feel your thighs relax. Your quads. Your core. Your buttocks. Breathe in. Feel the tension melt away as you continue to breath.

Feel the tension in your chest, in your shoulders, relax as you breath in and out. Breathe in and feel all the tension in your neck release. Feel the tension in your face, your forehead, your scalp relax as you continue to breathe. Breathe in and breathe out. Breathe in and breathe out. Feel all the tension in your wrists, your hands, your arms all the way up to your biceps and shoulders relax. Focus on your breathing and continue until you feel your entire body is completely relaxed.

Next, in your mind, I want you to go back to your childhood home. You're a grown person who is safe, travelling like you're like a ghost that can see and feel the home the way you did when you were a child.

Look around the home. What does the home look like? What color is it inside and out? What does it smell like? What does it sound like? What voices do you hear? What noises are there in your home? Who lives there? Who's there all the time? I want you to see the people moving through the house. What do they look like? What are they wearing? What do they smell like? What are they doing? I want you to experience what that place was really like.

See yourself in the home as a child, really zoom in and picture yourself as a child. What do you see? What do you look like? What are you wearing? What are you doing?

Now, one by one, I want you to take each person who's there and I want you to focus in on them. See them now as a grown-up looking at them. What do you see? Are they healthy? Are they fit? Are they overweight? Are they sick? What do they look like? What did they do for themselves? What did their actions towards themselves and others teach you? Did they work hard and never get good sleep or self-care, or did they make time for fun and relaxation? Did they show you what it was like to live a healthy balanced life? Did they teach you how to be healthy or unhealthy? To put yourself first or last, or not even on the list? Did your guardian take time every day to read or to pray or to meditate or to take a bath or to do something for themselves? Did they work from morning till night and pass out exhausted? Were they calm and peaceful or were they anxious or depressed or stressed or angry? What did you learn about self-care and health from that person either by what they said or about what they did?

See the message they gave you about self-care and health by how they treated themselves and by what they said to you. What did they say to you? Did they tell you to always take care of yourself and put yourself first? Did they tell you are important and you deserve love for who you are through words or by how they treated you? Did you get the message I'm only important by what I do for other people either the family or others? I'm only important if I get good grades. Do

I have to earn love or am I loved for who I am? What did you learn about yourself and what did you learn about health from that person?

I want you to move to the next person in the home. I want you to do the same observation about their habits and what they said and did around you, and what messages you got about yourself, health, and self-care from them. Look at that person and ask, how did they treat their bodies? What did you learn about health from them by how they treated themselves? What did you learn about how you should treat yourself and your own value by what they said or did to you? See the message you got from them. What is the stamp they put on you by what they did and what they said? Go to each person in your home and see them through your adult eyes. You are safe. You are a grown person. There's nothing that can hurt you in that space now. Just look at each person in the house, really look at them, and see what they taught you by what they did or what they said about how you should treat yourself. What did you learn from that home?

Finally, I want you to turn towards yourself as a child. I want you to see that child. How did he or she feel in that home? Did he or she feel loved and accepted and supported and taken care of and safe? Or did he or she feel unaccepted, unloved, unworthy, not good enough, ignored, alone? Did he or she feel empowered to achieve their dreams, or like a failure?

Now, I want you to sit down across from him or her and I want you to take his or her hand in your hand. I want you to look that child in the eyes. I want you to feel what that child feels and I want you to let them know that you are here now, and that you love that child for who that child is. You love them how they are. I want you to tell that child with all of your heart how much you love them. I want you to tell them you're sorry you weren't always there for them, that you didn't put them first, that you didn't take care of them the way they deserve. I want you to tell them you're sorry, that sometimes you put other priorities ahead of them. Really look in that child's eyes and tell them. And now I want you to tell them that from now on you will take amazing care of them. That you're not mad at them for not being what you wish they would be, that you don't resent them for not doing more, that you know that they are perfect and beautiful and deserve love and the best care, and that you will take such good care of them from now on.

You will give them the best food, you will let them take breaks, you will exercise their bodies so they can be strong and fit, you will do everything you can to make sure that child always feels loved, safe, important and taken care of from now on and for always. I want you to hold that child now. I want you to take that child in your arms and hold them and let them feel your commitment you'll always be there for them. Tell them again how you will take such good care of them and you will never judge them again and you will never make them feel unimportant or unloved or not good enough. You will do everything you can to make sure that that child always feels important. You will take care of them.

I want you to leave the house now. Walk out of the house. Stand in front of it and see it. And now I want you to close your eyes in your vision. Now you're in a place where you just feel safe and warm. You look up and you just see a bright warm light coming towards you. It's just feels like peace and love and you see it coming towards you and you stand there and you put your arms out and your head up and you feel the warmth of the light as it comes towards you closer and closer until it surrounds you. You feel safe and you feel pure love and light and safety. You're safe and you are loved. I want you to know that anytime you need to, you can come back to this place of love and light. I want you to breathe in and just feel it. Feel the warmth around you. Take it in. In this warm beautiful place, you know that you are strong and you are powerful. You know that all that you want is possible, and you can manifest it into your life by taking action every day. You can have health, you can have love, you can have safety, and it all comes from you. You can pull this light around you any time. Know that your health and your healing all comes from a place of love and light.

When you are ready, I want you to feel yourself coming back into your body again. Feel the chair or the bed or wherever you're sitting against the back of your legs and back. Feel the way your lungs expand and move your back against the surface you're leaning against. Feel your body again. When you're ready, you can open your eyes and come back. Take some deep breaths. Come back to this moment as you're ready. Know that being sick or being tired, none of that is your fault. None of that is your fault. Everything you are today comes from everything you learned growing up. This is not to place blame, but merely to understand. You can choose the lessons you want to keep from your childhood, and release the thoughts, beliefs, and habits that don't serve you. You can take care of yourself now. You can put yourself first. Whatever you think of yourself as an adult, remember that child is still in you. That child deserves amazing health and an amazing life. That child deserves at least fifteen minutes of your day to meditate or to exercise. It's your choice now to be that parent to yourself. If you find yourself struggling to do this for yourself, do it for that innocent child who deserves a health happy life. If you found this to be a powerful exercise, I encourage you to get a childhood photograph of yourself and place it somewhere visible, so you can tell the child in the photo every day that you love him or her and you will take great care of him or her today and every day from now on.

Assignment:

Write down what you saw during this exercise, the messages you received, both positive and negative, and your dedication to yourself to let go of past messages that don't serve you anymore and start taking the best care of yourself.

Chapter 23
You Don't Really See With Your Eyes

Did you know you don't see with your eyes? Most people think the information from your eyes tells your brain what you see, but that is not true. You actually see with your brain. Your eyes have optic nerves that travel all along the bottom of your brain to all the way back into the back of your brain, called the occipital lobe. The optic nerves sends an enormous amount of information, and your occipital lobe in your brain takes all the information coming from your eyes and filters out what it decides is extraneous and unimportant, and that is then relayed to your conscious mind as what you actually see. Thus, your brain decides what to let you see, it tells you what it thinks is important for you.

Have you ever been driving along a road you have been down many times before and suddenly noticed something you never saw before? Then you find out it has always been there, but you didn't see it. Why didn't you notice it before? The truth is, you did see it with your eyes. You saw the object every time you drove by. Your brain just filtered out the information because it decided it wasn't important to you. Then one day, that detail got through and you saw it, seemingly for the first time. Fascinating, isn't it?

That is the same way our emotional minds work. We receive a lot of input every single day. Our mind decides what we experience. Our mind decides what we see. If you're used to seeing things negatively, if you're used to seeing pain and loss, then even when things are going great your mind will look for pain and loss. If that is your mindset, then no matter how much healing you are experiencing, your mind will filter out the good and focus on the bad. You will only see negatives. If you want to change that, you need to create a new mental habit where you embrace the good things instead of the bad. Look for the good things every day. That way, any negative information just becomes a little bit of information and not your entire view point. That is why I teach you to count your celebrations every day, because if you are in the habit of filtering out the good, I want you to look for it, tell your mind that it is important so you can start seeing all your wins. You need to tell your brain to expand your view: notice and embrace all the positives coming in. Tell your brain you want to see more; you want to see differently. Notice things you never noticed before.

So, focus on celebrations as part of your recovery. If you're not focusing on your celebrations, you miss out on how much better you are. If you focus on negative, you're robbing yourself of your recovery and happiness. If you notice negativity creeping in, tell your brain "I want to see more." I want to see all the beauty around me and in me. There are so many great things happening in your body and all around you. Remind your brain you want to see it. You deserve to see it.

Chapter 24
Dealing With Cravings

When you are getting off of the foods you're addicted to, your body will scream and shout and have a tantrum. That is because you are in physical withdrawal from the most addictive and destructive drug on the planet, junk foods. The foods you're addicted to, whether they're cooked, whether it's oily foods, dairy or meat, create a physical high in your body that food was never meant to create. You literally get a rush of dopamine from oils, sugars, and meats beyond the level you can ever get from whole healthy plant foods. We're not supposed to get high on food. The reason that eating releases any dopamine at all is because we're supposed to be physiologically pulled to eat; eating healthy food gives of a small dose of dopamine as a reward to do that activity. It keeps us alive. Unfortunately, once you expose the brain to unhealthy foods it is difficult to stop consuming them.

In western countries processed foods and animal products have become a primary source of food intake, causing not just chronic deadly diseases, but emotional misery. Unhealthy food has become so addictive that many people are using it as a source of happiness rather than something we need as fuel. The dopamine release from unhealthy food is so powerful, that other activities that create dopamine like exercise and physical contact are not sought out. People depend on food for their highs.

There was an experiment once on rats where the scientists gave them a choice between food and cocaine. When given that choice, the rat chooses the cocaine exclusively and eventually dies.[20] The cocaine stimulated their brain and made them feel more high than eating, therefore the drive to use cocaine superseded the drive to eat. Humans have done this too, but instead of using cocaine, we created cocaine-like food. People are choosing to eat things that kill them—pizza and burgers and French fries and soda, while they simultaneously malnourish themselves of vitamins and minerals and water. Humans eat foods that kill them instead of eating foods that heal them. It's an addiction. So, when someone says, "I would love to get my health back, but I love cheese too much to stop eating it," I educate them that they do not, in fact, love cheese, they are addicted to it. And that addiction is killing them. That is often a wakeup call that starts a deeper more open conversation.

The only way to reverse addiction and cravings is to stop eating the food you're addicted to. There's no other way around it. As long as you have even a little bit of cocaine, you will be addicted to cocaine. To stop a drug addiction, you need to go through the withdrawal process. It's the same with food. You need to go through withdrawal and detoxification from the unhealthy food. In the beginning that might mean healthy foods will not taste great. They will feel boring or unfulfilling. That's not because they're not good for you. It's because you're not getting a high from eating them.

So, what do you do in the meantime? You need to learn how to get high another way that is healthy for you. That is why self-care is so important. You need to get in the habit of using activities and relationships to feel good, not food. The activities that provide the greatest source of dopamine are high-intensity exercise, sexual activity, and spending time with friends that make you feel happy. There is also dopamine upregulation from getting enough sleep, listening to music, and meditation.

If you feel stressed, don't comfort yourself with food, use meditation, listening to beautiful music, going for walks in nature, take long luxurious baths, and other relaxing activities to soothe your senses and help you feel more peaceful.

The clients I have that have conquered food addictions the fastest used a combination of these activities: a daily self-care routine for relaxation like meditation, at least 5 minutes a day of high intensity exercise most days of the week, like high intensity interval cardio or boot camp style workouts, and getting at least 7 hours of sleep a night.

Inflammatory foods are one of the most powerful drugs around. They're also one of the most deadly. If you're looking for a salad that is going to give you a high like pizza, it is just not possible. What you need to do is get high off life and stop looking for food to make you happy. Create happiness through your experiences and relationships and stop wanting your food to be your emotional partner. You've got to want your health more than you want to get high.

If you find yourself thinking, "I miss the foods I love," remind yourself that those foods don't love you back. Think of those foods you think you love as a cruel ex that abused you. Don't keep going back to an abusive partner. You've got to start a new relationship with food that's healthy.

Chapter 25
Stop Anxiety Before It Stops You

What I found over the years is that many people with chronic diseases have the same symptoms I saw in my mental health patients that survived trauma. Chronic disease and trauma patients often have that same fear for their lives and a sense of impending doom, the same constant worry, and agitation. Post-traumatic stress disorder is caused by an event or events that makes the person feel like his or her life is in danger, or witnessing someone else almost or actually die. The most common analogy is a soldier coming home from war. I also saw it in patients that grew up in gang neighborhoods seeing people getting shot on their streets, or victims of physical or sexual abuse. Getting diagnosed with a disease can create trauma as well, as you face your own mortality. Also, studies have shown that people who are survivors of trauma are far more likely to develop autoimmune disease later, causality being linked to the stress on the body creating chronic inflammation that triggers their illnesses.[21] Thus, whether anxiety precipitated the illness, or the illness caused the anxiety, it is very common to have both chronic illness and chronic anxiety, and we need to address both if they coexist to help you eliminate inflammation and disease.

These techniques are not meant to replace seeing a great therapist, going to a psychiatrist and getting the help and support you need. If you're dealing with terrible depression, anxiety, or negativity, you need to get the right help. I find trauma specialists are a good idea if you don't have somebody to talk to yet.

First, I want to teach you a quick technique to use when you're having a lot of anxiety or panic.

This technique will help you control the panic or anxiety. It's simple.

1. Take a deep breath through your nose.
2. Hold it for a second, before breathing out through your nose.
3. Every time you breathe in, say your first name in your head. Repeat this a few times.

4. Then, think of one word to describe how you want to feel. Some examples are safe, loved, or peace. Think of one or at most two words to describe how you want to feel.

5. Breathe in, think your name; Breathe out, think your mood word(s).

This tackles the anxiety on two levels: first because anxious brains like to be busy and you're giving it an activity to do that does not cause anxiety. You're not thinking bad, worrisome stuff. You're just breathing and thinking your name and mood. Second, this technique is also a type of self-hypnosis. You anchor that mood with your name. If you say your name and that mood repeatedly, it causes a state of mild hypnosis where you create that mood for yourself in the moment. I've used this technique to bring people down from panic attacks in the clinics. It's even better to use it before you're panicking. If you're already starting to notice you're getting more anxious, take a break, do this technique and let yourself calm down. You can try different words to see what resonates the most but pick something that feels like what you're looking to feel. It's got to be a mood. It's not something physical you want, but how you want to feel. You can do this exercise any time you feel anxious. It's simple and works really well. It's also a great practice to start your day with this exercise.

Another technique to help anxiety is using a thought log. This is a technique derived from cognitive behavioral therapy. When you feel anxious or upset, identify the thought that is triggering your mood and work on it. For example, let's say the thought is "I'll never get better", instead of sitting there with the negativity and fear hanging over you, use this technique to dislodge the thought and improve your mood.

1. Describe the situation that triggered your low mood and negative thoughts. What's going on right now that's making you feel unhappy. What's triggering the thought you're having. What are you doing? What time of day is it? What's happening that triggered the thought? In this example, maybe you feel more pain today.
2. Identify and rate your mood. How do you feel? Are you sad, hopeless, depressed? Write a percentage next to it. Maybe you're 50% sad, 60% hopeless, 70% depressed, etc.

3. Identify the thoughts or images that come to your head. If you're having the thought "I'll never get better" write that down. Sometimes it's not so much a thought, but an image like you lying in bed or you never enjoying your life. Whatever it is, write it down.
4. Write down facts that support my thought. Why do you think this thought or image is true? Have you been sick for ten years and still have symptoms? Does everyone in your family die of chronic illness? There are real reasons for you to have these thoughts, this is where you list them. Write the facts, not thoughts or fears, but facts.
5. Write down facts that do not support my thought. If you can't think of anything to write, ask yourself what someone who had positive thinking would say. Use that to come up with evidence against your negative thoughts. When you feel depressed, it's hard to come up with positive things, but it's very important that you work hard to find evidence against what you're thinking. If you are struggling on your own, think about what a positive friend or support person in your life would tell you. Examples: "A bad day doesn't mean I am not getting better," "thousands of people have gotten their health back this way and I am made of the same human parts that they are," "I have a lot more energy than I did before".
6. Create a balanced new thought to replace the original negative thought. You will take your original thought you wrote in number three and rewrite it using the evidence you wrote in four and five, taking into consideration the evidence for and against your negative thoughts. You don't just want to write the opposite thought, because your mind won't believe it. Your mind came up with this thought based on its own evidence, and it won't accept being shut down completely. Rather, aim for a thought that takes negatives and positives into account, so it is more balanced. For example, if the original thought was "I will never heal" then the balance thought, based on the evidence we just said, would be, "Although I still have symptoms and people in my family are all ill, I have witnessed through other people's testimonials that this can really work, and I have already experienced better energy, which shows I am improving."

You see this is not 100% positive, it just moves you from the all negative, to a place that is more in the middle between positive and negative. People's minds are less likely to reject a new thought like that, than they are a totally opposite thought.

7. Rate your emotions now. Maybe sad went from 50% to 40%. Maybe anxious went from 70% to 30.% Maybe depressed went from 70% to 20%. Write how you feel now.

Thoughts, feelings, and behaviors are all linked to each other. When you're having negative thoughts, you will have more negative feelings. When you have negative thoughts and feelings, you are more likely to take negative actions against yourself, like quitting or eating off plan, or neglecting self-care of exercise. While it is very hard to change a feeling, working on thoughts can be very productive. If you can just go from a 100% negative thought to a thought that's more balanced, you can have a positive impact in your mood right there. I encourage you to try these techniques. By taking steps like this, as well as seeking the right counseling, you can improve your health all the way around.

PART FIVE
CASE STUDIES

"While data and science are interesting, it's real people's stories of recovery that inspire us the most. Thank you to every person who honored me by choosing me as your guide and your coach to get your health back.

Some people willingly shared their first and last names, some requested just their first name, and others have had their names changed for privacy. All of them have amazing stories of recovery, and I hope they inspire you to follow in their footsteps."

Dr. G

Chapter 26
Case Study #1: Debbie's* Story

> *Rheumatoid Arthritis: Going From a Standard American Diet to High Raw Recovery Diet*

Every person I helped heal from disease who lives their lives again, changes my life too. But don't just take my word for it. I want them to tell you their stories in their own words.

The first person I want to introduce you to is Debbie. I met Debbie because she ran into my mother at a furniture store. My mom is the kind of person that, if you meet her, you tell her your whole life story. Debbie ended up telling my mom about her rheumatoid arthritis and mom said 'oh, you need to meet my daughter.' She made an appointment with me and I created a personalized nutrition plan for her to reverse her disease.

Debbie had severe pain in her legs, ranging from eight to ten out of ten by the end of the day. She came home from work exhausted and didn't have energy to play with her kids. She was an avid runner and loved exercise, but could no longer run on her arthritic knees. She was on oral medications and injections of anti-inflammatory medicine into her knees every week, and this was the best medication could do for her.

When I do a private consultation over the phone, via facetime or a video meeting online, I spend sixty to seventy-five minutes with the client to get to know their story, understand their symptoms and their goals, and analyze their current diet. Then I take their current diet and I show them how to make step by step improvements to optimize their recovery. I help them identify which essential foods they are missing, the inflammatory foods they need to eliminate, and how to convert their current diet into a similar one that is made of unprocessed plant foods and healing nutrition. I also teach them how they can do more aggressive approaches that consists of 75% or greater raw healing foods to accelerate their recovery. I also address any issues I see with motivation, stress, sleep or other areas of their lifestyle that might be creating inflammation.

Debbie was relatively happy outside of her disease: she has a supportive husband, enjoys being a mother, and doesn't carry a lot of stress outside of her pain. Her diet was the main source of inflammation and disease causing and exacerbating her disease.

This was Debbie's Diet before we met - see if you can identify the inflammatory foods and the healing foods. If you need a review, check out section VII after the introduction in this book, or refer to detailed explanations in the book Goodbye Lupus.

Breakfast: oatmeal, fruit, a protein shake, eggs, and an English muffin for breakfast.

Lunch: Lean Cuisine

Snacks, carrots, roasted nuts, a lot of protein bars, apples, and string cheese.

Dinner. "Heavy Italian Foods", quinoa, broccoli rabe cooked in oil, salmon and chicken cooked in oil, meatballs, and sausage.

Water: 64 ounces a day

Analysis:

Breakfast:

Inflammatory: eggs (animal product), English muffin (processed), whey protein shake (animal products and processed).

Neutral: Oatmeal, fruit

Anti-inflammatory: None

Lunch:

Inflammatory: Lean Cuisine (The inflammatory trifecta: processed, oils, animal products)

Neutral: None

Anti-inflammatory: None.

Snacks:

Inflammatory: protein bars (animal products, processed), string cheese (animal products), roasted nuts (oils)

Neutral: apples

Anti-inflammatory: carrots - I will give this one to her. They are the best choice if they are whole carrots. Baby carrots are skinned and bleached and offer very little nutrition compared to whole carrots with the mineral-rich skin.

Dinner:

Inflammatory: Salmon, meatballs, and chicken (animal products, oil), broccoli rabe (oil),

Neutral: Quinoa

Anti-inflammatory: I will give some credit for the Broccoli, however since it was cooked it had very little anti-inflammatory power left.

Summary:

Very high in inflammatory foods, and as for the anti-inflammatory components that she needs:

- Very low in water (less than 96 ounces a day),
- Very low in omega-3s (maybe small amount from fish if it were wild caught, but omega 3s are heat sensitive and fish also has omega-6 and saturated fats so still very low to no daily intake),
- Very low raw vegetable intake, no raw leafy greens or cruciferous on a daily basis.

Most people would look at this diet and think it's relatively healthy, but it's actually an inflammatory diet. I told Debbie, "Good news! Your diet is making you sick, we can fix it." We changed her breakfast to green smoothies made from 75% greens, ½ cup of flax or chia seeds, water, and 25% fruit for breakfast. Snacks were now either fresh fruit, a handful of raw nuts, or broccoli with guacamole. Dinner was a big salad or quinoa with steamed vegetables. She could still have dessert, but no dairy ice cream or whipped cream. Dessert was now frozen bananas with a splash of almond milk mixed into a soft serve ice cream in her blender. Plus, we increased Debbie's water intake from 64 ounces a day to a 128 ounces, which is a gallon or 3.8 liters a day.

One week after our appointment, she sent me a text message saying she felt so good she was literally skipping in a parking lot! I'd like to let you hear Debbie's story in her own words.

> "Hi my name is Debbie*, I'm a 45 year old woman and I have rheumatoid arthritis. I was diagnosed about two years ago, very rapidly my range of motion and my ability to do the things that I used to do decline, I was in pain and uncomfortable and just unhappy. I also have two little girls that are six and seven and I went from running with them in a double jogging stroller to barely being able to sit on the floor and play with them. I was on a couple different pills methotrexate, doing the shots, one in each leg every week and just wasn't feeling any better. By happenstance I found Dr. Goldner and I did exactly what she told me to do. Not only did I start feeling better in the first week, but I was off all of my medications within three weeks. I can't believe it, it's awesome. It's been four months now that I am following her program and I feel awesome. I'm completely off the medications, I am working out in the yard every day planting and digging and gardening and doing whatever...I'm an artist and I'm on my feet a lot and I don't know when to stop and I'm able to have more stamina and to do more of what I need to do.
>
> So, thanks to Dr. Goldner, I am a better mother hopefully, I am a hard-working person, I'm a better artist, I am a gardener and I am back to being the person that I used to be, so thanks Doc."
>
> *Name has been changed to protect identity

Chapter 27
Case Study#2: Carla's* Story

> *Lupus: Going from a High Starch Low Fat Plant-Based Diet to Full Rapid Recovery Diet*

The next person I'd like to introduce you to is Carla who was diagnosed with Lupus. Her symptoms were so severe, she planned to go on disability. She couldn't function anymore. Her rheumatologist was aware of the power of plant-based nutrition to help reverse diseases, and put her on a plant-based diet that consisted of cooked vegetables, potatoes, beans, and no added fats. However, after a few months on a plant-based diet, Carla did not have significant changes in her pain levels or energy. She still could not get out of a chair and stand up on her own without pushing on the arms of the chair with her hands to push herself up. She could not bend down to put on her pants, and instead had to use a claw tool to bring her pants up her legs. Her legs were so weak and painful, she had not been able to climb stairs in 2 years. This affected her work, because she was supposed to lead a weekly meeting at work that was up 2 flights of stairs and she had been unable to make it there. This was one reason she thought that leaving work on disability was her only option. She was exhausted and struggled to get to work by 9:00am, and still found herself falling asleep by 7:00pm in the evening. She didn't have the energy to enjoy her relationship, walk her dogs, or do anything else besides work and rest, and she no longer felt she was productive at the job she loved. When the change to a plant-based diet didn't help her heal, her doctor suggested Carla do my 4 week rapid recovery program before giving up and quitting her job. She called me to set it up as her last hope.

Carla followed my program to the T. No inflammatory foods, no cooked foods, just healing foods consisting of raw vegetables, especially dark leafy greens and cruciferous vegetables, high omega-3s from flax or chia, and she drank a gallon of water every day. She wanted to heal herself and take back her life.

I want to show you her case in more detail so you can see what it looks like when someone is actually on the rapid recovery program. On day four she already had dramatically decreased pain, increased mobility, and increased energy. She wrote to me, "Great day, pain would be a 0.5! I am just so excited that I have more energy, and don't hurt. Makes walking the dogs easier, cleaning the house, and walking around at work." It was only 4 days after changing her diet from traditional cooked plant foods to hyper-nourishing raw foods and high omega-3s and water, and her pain was almost gone and she was productive at work and when she got home. She was already happy with her results and she had just gotten started.

By day six, she already had full range of motion in her legs and hips, which she discovered when she found herself having to change flat tires. She wrote to me on day 6, "Energy was good today. Two flat tires today…so I had the opportunity to complete repairs. I was uncomfortable, but was able to tolerate the job. It is amazing the decrease in symptoms I noticed yesterday." This is the same woman who couldn't even bend down to put her own pants on six days ago!

On day eight, Carla reported, "Mild stiffness in A.M., but it is gone by 11 A.M. Today's a good day. No discomfort in quads when walking up hill." She was not only going for walks, she was taking the hills and feeling no pain! If all this was achieved with a pill, it would be ground-breaking and the number one pill on the market. There would be talks of Nobel prizes. But this was not a new medication, Carla achieved these results by drinking green smoothies with ingredients she got at her local supermarket. Amazing, right?

By day ten, Carla's rheumatologist started tapering her off her steroids. When she came to me 10 days prior, her meds weren't giving her any relief. Now she was pain free and coming down off her medications, again with only dietary intervention. She wrote to me. "My Rheumatologist started tapering my steroids! I can walk without feeling like I am wearing cement shoes. I walked up the hill today and didn't even think about it. I was able to go a short bike ride of about 2 miles. I have not ridden a bike in over 1 year!"

On day thirteen, I got this incredible life-changing message. "I can walk up and down stairs!" After 2 years of being unable to use the stairs, and thinking this disability would keep her from the job she loved, she was now fully mobile again. Less than 2 weeks after changing her diet, she was pain free and e energetic, and no longer experienced the restrictions and loss that years with lupus had caused her.

On day twenty-one, her energy was at an all-time high, she wrote, "I can stay awake till 10:30-11:00 pm! Pleased with the weight loss also (8lbs), but not as much as I am pleased with an increase in my energy."

On day twenty-four I was shocked and delighted to receive this message from Carla, "Able to work for 2 hours with splitting wood; I was sore for about an hour after. Not bad." One of the things I admire most about Carla is that she was chomping at the bit to get back to living at 100%. The better she felt, the more she did. She went from barely moving besides dragging herself to work and back home every day to walking, hiking, biking, and even chopping wood. She relished and embraced her newfound vitality and didn't waste a moment getting back to her full life. I have found over the years doing rapid recovery programs that folks who move as soon as they are able, exercising and doing activities they love and enjoy, have accelerated recovery time. That is why I include self-care and exercise in the program now. Carla did this automatically, and every day was dramatically better than the day before.

By the last day, day twenty-eight, Carla reported that she was under 200lbs for the first time in her adult life. In 4 weeks, she had changed her life in every way. At that point, she no longer planned to retire, instead she was planning travel. She decided to marry her long-time partner, who had been her caretaker when she was sick, and she sent me photographs of them hiking the Grand Canyon together on their honeymoon.

This is why I do this work, whether I am seeing people for appointments online, holding people's hands every day with my Rapid Recovery programs, teaching or writing, my goal is to help everyone I can live a life without pain and disease, and more importantly, a life with love and purpose and joy, just like Carla.

After the 4 Week Rapid Recovery Program was complete, Carla was ready for step-down, where she added back foods like beans and cooked vegetables, while continuing to hyper-nourish with green smoothies full of dark leafy greens and omega-3s every day, maintaining high water intake of 96 to 128 ounces a day. She continued to be pain free and energetic. When I checked in with her 7 months later, she emailed me this:

> "Still no joint pain (YAY)… Folks from work and my bible study group have asked me to share my green drink because they have noticed the weight loss and the overall health benefits. Staying as close as I can to plant-based living is also better for me. Have I been totally vegan? No. I have had beef, venison, fish, and cheese probably on 7-10 occasions since I started the lupus program… I could tell my body was unhappy with that choice… I am back to eating green."

Carla's case demonstrates that while it took the strictest totally raw vegan diet to reverse her illness, now that she is healthy she can incorporate cooked plant foods and even the occasional animal-based food and maintain her health. Now she does feel tired and sick to her stomach when she eats animal foods, as she notes her body is "unhappy with that choice", but she does not get a lupus flare-up. When your body is used to clean fuel, you feel less vibrant and often get gastrointestinal upset when you try to eat inflammatory foods like processed foods, oily foods, or animal-based foods, but if you listen to that signal from your body and get back to the good foods, it won't progress back to chronic illness again.

Now I have seen people get autoimmune symptoms back again from adding back inflammatory foods too quickly after their initial recovery, before their disease was fully reversed. For that reason, I recommend that if you do plan to eat inflammatory foods on occasion, make sure you have been completely symptom-free and healthy for 6 months or greater to ensure you are truly fully recovered and don't, in essence, rip the scab off of a healing wound when you are in the early stages of recovery and disease reversal but not fully recovered.

* Name changed to protect identity

Chapter 28
Case Study#3: Danielle's Story

Lupus & Sjogren's: From Standard American Diet to Full Rapid Recovery Nutrition Protocol

Danielle came to me diagnosed with Lupus and Sjogren's. She was referred to me by the Director of Neurology at her local hospital. At the time she was 29 years old. Her symptoms were very severe. She had dry, burning eyes, dry mouth, chronic arthritis, hair loss, butterfly rash and neuropathy in both hands. Sometimes her hands fell asleep while driving. She experienced light headiness, blurred vision and exhaustion from severe photosensitivity or sensitivity to light. Simply walking to her car would trigger an episode. Her exhaustion was off the charts.

She suffered from debilitating pleurisy which brought her to the emergency room several times and caused her to miss her college graduation ceremony. Keeping up with a social life was challenging because of all the pain and exhaustion she was struggling with. While her rheumatologist told her that medications were the treatment, and was unsure how to help her feel better, her neurologist told her about me and encouraged her to try using nutrition to reverse her symptoms. She was eager to begin and made a phone appointment to get started right away.

Danielle was dedicated and eager, and her results reflected her high commitment level. She had regular phone appointments with me to adjust her diet as needed, and addressed obstacles she faced. She became interested in fun raw recipes, and started blogging about her progress to inspire others. Her neuropathy disappeared in 2 weeks, rapidly followed by pain melting away and energy through the roof.

Her photosensitivity also disappeared, and she now enjoys being outside without layers of clothing and a big hat to protect her. Not only that, she went on multiple Caribbean cruises and was out in the sun all day and still felt great! I celebrated this with her whole-heartedly. One of the most freeing experiences for me when I healed from Lupus was being able to be out in the sunlight like other people. I lived like a vampire for 12 years because the sun would cause pain and rashes and extreme fatigue, and when I healed I spent every free moment soaking in the warm rays of the sun. I still do. Seeing Danielle out and about enjoying the sunshine again gave me tremendous joy.

In the years since we first met, Danielle has remained disease-free and active, and even gotten married. She lives a full active life and enjoys inspiring people on Instagram @SproutBelly with her story of recovery and delicious recipes. Of note, Danielle had a full reversal of her symptoms before her labs responded in kind. I remember having a session with her 6 months after she had been completely symptoms free. She was running outside, lifting weights, feeling energetic and pain-free, and very happy. Then she got her labs drawn and while the majority were completely normal and indicated no illness at all, her anti-DSDNA antibodies were still positive. They were down from previously, but not gone. She got upset and questioned her recovery. I reminded her that people often feel sick for years before their labs become positive, and sometimes it takes many months of being healthy before the labs are fully normal again, but that doesn't mean you are not better. The better way to judge how healthy you are is by how you feel. She admitted she felt amazing. I told her we would never normally test the anti-DSDNA antibodies of a healthy person running around feeling amazing!

Antibodies have their own life span, and while some people find their antibodies come down quickly, others have a slow and steady decline in antibodies while all the other signs of acute inflammation like complement and sedimentation rate and C-Reactive Protein normalize more rapidly

Here is what Danielle had to say about her recovery the year we met.

> Hi my name is Danielle, I'm 29 years old and I was diagnosed with lupus and Sjogren's. I was extremely sensitive to sunlight, I would consistently get sick with the butterfly rash, and tunnel vision. I developed joint stiffness in my fingers, my elbows and my knees. I had pleurisy which was very painful and all led me to the emergency room. I was napping and sleeping all the time. My mouth was so dry and I developed dry eyes. My arms would go numb, my fingers would tingle

driving. I saw a neurologist; he said he knew a doctor that had lupus and that she didn't have lupus anymore, she healed herself through her nutrition protocol, and I was all about it!

So immediately I followed her protocol. The time and patience she put into teaching how to care for myself was invaluable. Within two weeks I could sit at my desk and type without my fingers feeling like there's needles in them. I could drive my car without my arms going numb. It was such a drastic change. The sun was a big one; this past weekend I went shopping in the sun, I wore a t-shirt and I did great! My butterfly rash wasn't there, no tunnel vision, no spots to blur my vision, and I don't suffer from stiff joints at all anymore. I am not tired. I have a renewed sense of energy. Now I run miles, I enjoy working out, I lift weights, I have energy to do this. I honestly don't know where I would be if the neurologist didn't mention Dr. Goldner to me, I am back to my normal self!

Chapter 29
Case Study #4: David's Bridges Story

Lupus, Scleroderma & Sjogren's: From Highly Processed Standard American Diet to Hyper-Nourishment With Minimal Animal Products.

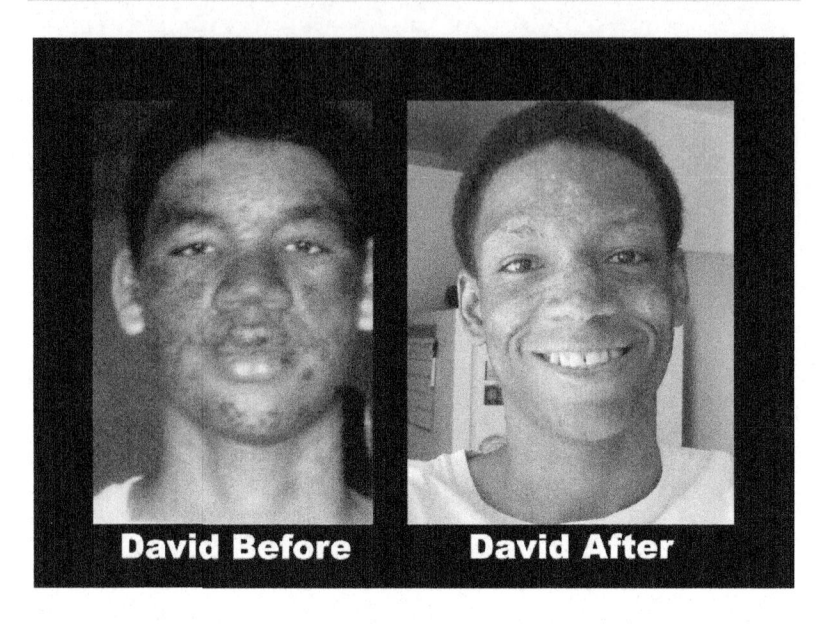

David Before   **David After**

David had lupus, Sjogren's, and scleroderma since he was 16-years-old. He spent as much as four months in the ICU at a time. The doctors told his mother Glenda repeatedly that she needed to say goodbye, that he wasn't going to make it. She is a single mom and he is her only child, and she would not give up. She constantly advocated for the best care possible, but sadly he was stick very sick and in pain, and he was not getting better.

Glenda works as a therapist, and he would stay home while she worked to support them. One day, I was invited to give a talk for therapists on nutrition and mental health. She had considered not going, but she needed the continuing education credits and decided to show up, without knowing anything about me or the topic being presented. While introducing myself, I talked about how I became aware of the power of nutrition to heal the body through my own recovery from lupus, and she lit up. She came up to me after the talk and told me "I've been praying for someone to help my David and I think you're the one." I promised to do everything I could to help. David became my first ever telemedicine disease-reversal patient.

David suffered from painful rashes on his face, swollen eyes, nose, and lips, edema in his legs. Scleroderma hardened his skin, which broke open at the joints of his fingers. The open wounds were constantly infected deep into his joints, causing excruciating pain when he tried to move or use his hands. He couldn't button his own shirt because his fingers were too stiff and painful. When Glenda asked his doctors what they could do to help his fingers, the only solution they offered was to amputate his fingertips. Can you imagine? In addition, he had a large red rash that covered his entire face, and parts of his scalp. His cheeks, nose, and lips were swollen. He had areas of hair loss or alopecia as well. His legs were swollen with edema. Between his swollen painful face and his swollen infected fingers, he told me that people had difficulty looking at him. In spite of constant chronic illness since the age of 15, he had managed to finish high school and get a degree from a community college, and yet he could not get a job. He told me he went on job interviews, hoping to work and be productive. He has a big heart and wanted a job where he could help others in need. He said that interviewers barely looked at him and he never got a job. David wanted to be seen, to be understood, to have purpose, and share his heart with others, and his illnesses were a barrier that kept him isolated, alone with his pain.

At the time, David was getting a lot of his food from 7-11 next door to his house, a market that sells basic home products and a lot of processed junk foods and soda. He said he made his own foods as well, but put "butter on everything". He added cheese to a lot of his meals as well. He ate very little vegetables (and what he did eat was slathered in butter) and no raw vegetables, no omega 3s, and little to no water. Unbeknownst to him or his mother, his diet was literally killing him.

After our first consult, David agreed to do hyper-nourishment, but was not ready to do the complete protocol. Essentially, he did everything but eliminate meat. He added in tons of greens, water, and omega-3s, and even eliminated butter and dairy, but still ate meat once a week. He drank about 90 ounces of green smoothie a day, made with 75% or more dark leafy greens like kale and spinach and mixed greens. He took in high doses of omega 3s and 128 ounces of water a day. Even though he had occasional meat, he started healing rapidly. His skin rash cleared up completely and all of his hair grew back except one little dime-sized spot that had scarred over but was easy to cover with his new growth of healthy hair. The infections in his hands cleared up and the skin on his joint healed and closed up. He could use his fingers again. A few short months later, he got a job as a case worker helping under-served youth in Los Angeles California. He was in remission. His symptoms had resolved, and his labs were dramatically better, but still positive. His doctors reduced his medication. He continued eating this way for 2 years and he remained in remission.

What David's story shows is if you're not ready to dive in all the way, adding what you're missing is an amazing start. Decrease inflammatory foods as you can. By hyper-nourishing, and minimizing inflammatory foods, David saw a dramatic improvement in his energy and mood, he barely had any pain in his joints. He could get a job which is the number one thing he told me he wanted before starting the program. His diseases were in remission, not gone because he decided not to do the full protocol, but in remission and he was living a full life without limitations.

Now for a lot of people this would be a welcome miracle. For those of you who are sick right now, wouldn't you love to have no symptoms and be on minimal medicines? Every step you take towards embracing the full hyper-nourishing nutrition protocol for disease reversal will get you healthier and closer to the health you want. If you hyper-nourish and you minimize the unhealthy foods, you can get dramatically better. You likely won't completely reverse your illness, but you can get dramatically better.

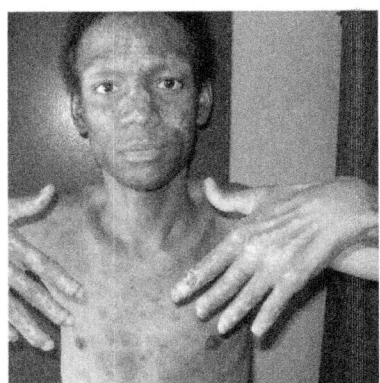

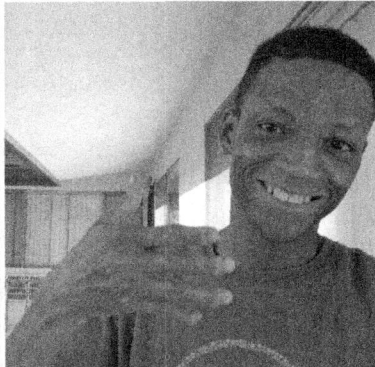

David Before   David After

This offers insight into why people with autoimmune disease can sometimes experience remission of symptoms with nutrition plans that include meat, like the currently popular "Paleo diet". It is not really representative of what Paleolithic humans ate, but attempts to imitate the more natural way of eating prior to the introduction of processed foods. Followers of this diet are told to eliminate dairy and processed foods, and focus on "free-range" meat and vegetables. Now for the majority of people out there, that is a drastic improvement in their nutrition over the standard highly processed and dairy-filled foods people typically eat. So, if you tend to like vegetables and you get rid of dairy and processed foods and just eat some meat on occasion, you're going to have a significant improvement in your health. Unfortunately, the people who tend to eat a lot of meat and fewer vegetables often get sicker. I have had multiple clients who came to me after trying "Paleo" who got severely ill. One developed lupus after eating chicken and eggs every meal multiple times a day while doing a combination of CrossFit workouts and "Paleo diet" given to her by her trainers. She lost a lot of weight, had 6-pack abs for the first time in her life, and had such bad arthritis she could no longer use her hands, ending up diagnosed with lupus. Two others who already had autoimmune disease went into kidney failure after eating a "Paleo diet" given to them by their healthcare providers. All of these people had rapid reversal of their illnesses on my plant-based protocol. I believe that a nutrition plan where some people get better and some people get much worse is not a good nutrition plan! Even with those that can achieve remission with a healthier version of a "Paleo" type plan, the disease is still there and can come back whenever they eat off plan.

When you get rid of all the foods that are making you sick, that's when the miracles happen.

As I mentioned, David was able to continue in remission on minimal medications for about two years before I saw him again. He and his mother stayed in touch with me over the years, sending me text messages when good things happen, and wishing me happy holidays. I was in Los Angeles with my husband Thomas, teaching a two-day conference called Amazing Fitness and health. I invited David and Glenda to attend and I was really excited to see them both. He looked so good! No more rashes, no more infections, no swollen legs! His hands have some deformity in their shape from years of infections in his bones, but they were healed up and he could use them.

During the conference I taught the 6 Steps to Healing With Supermarket Foods and he had a revelation. He had forgotten about my recommendations to not eat meat. He decided to give up the meat and stick to a 100% plant-based diet. He would eat beans and cooked vegetables, and his big blenders of nourishing raw vegetables and omega 3s, high water intake, and he would see if he could take his health to the next level.

Within days after completely eliminating all animal products, he checks in with me and says the skin is glowing now. A couple weeks later, he texts me that his joints felt "super flexible". Then, 2 months later, I get this text from his mother:

> "Guess what? David's rheumatologist is taking him off all of his medications."

So, with doing most of the program but still eating some meat he was able to get remission of his symptoms and maintain his health on a very low dose of medicines. Once he committed a hundred percent to this program and eliminated meat as well, he was able to come off all of his medicines and continue to be healthy. It has been over 4 years since this happened, and he continues to be 100% symptom free, with normal labs and no medications.

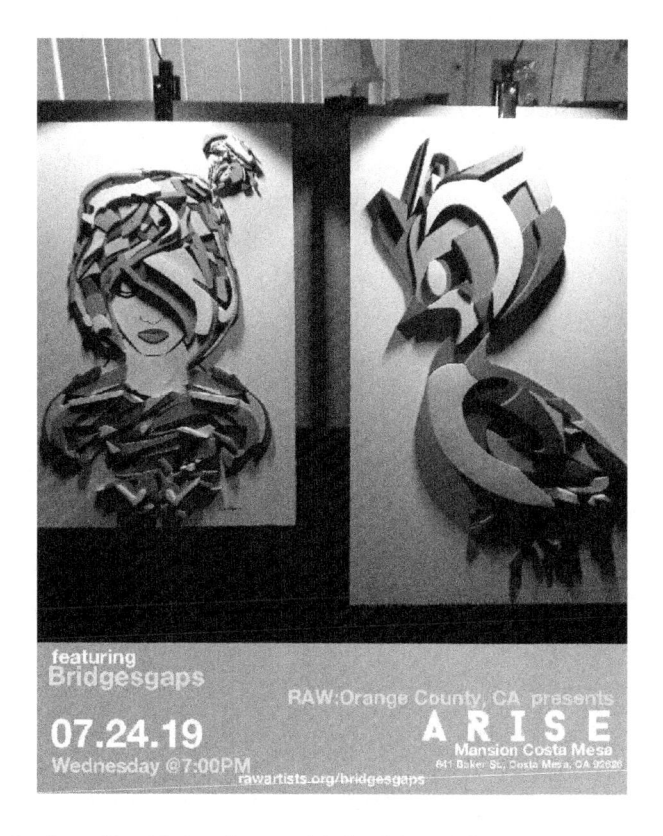

When you look at David, he glows with health and happiness. He has gotten 2 promotions at work and now has people working under him. He teaches his clients about good mental health and exercise and eating healthy. He told me that they affectionately call him the rabbit at work and they gave him a big bunch of carrots for his birthday. He loved it. He also started creating incredible 3-dimensional art and has been featured in Galleries around Los Angeles. Not that long ago, his hands hurt so badly he couldn't hold a paint brush, doctors were planning to amputate his fingers, and now he is an up and coming artist. The world was almost deprived of his immense gifts. David also has fallen in love and is currently planning his wedding.

His mother Glenda carries my book Goodbye Lupus in her purse along with before-and-after pictures of David, because constantly she meets people who are sick and suffering and she wants to inspire them to take their lives back the way her David did.

It means so much to me it means so much to me to help people like David to go from being sick and in pain and alone, with no hope or purpose or passion in their lives, to becoming pain and symptom free, working, loving, creating art, and living with passion and joy. It's what I want for you too. That's the difference, that's the difference that the right nutrition can make, and unlike other ways of eating, these results are typical, you can have results like this too.

Chapter 30
Case Study #5: Emily Horowitz's Story

> *Sjogren's and Lupus: From "Mostly Vegan" with Expensive Supplements To Rapid Recovery*

Emily Horowitz came to me with lupus and Sjogren's. She was a 46 years old college professor and had severe dry eyes and mouth, and chronic itching on her scalp. Her ophthalmologist said her eyes were "very dry and inflamed." She also had joint pain "in all joints", especially her hips. Her doctor said she would need a hip replacement surgery. She also had numbness in her fingers and toes. She first thought there were other explanations for her symptoms. She had constant gut irritation and thought she had Irritable Bowel. She was an avid writer, and blamed her wrist and finger pain on Carpal Tunnel syndrome from excessive typing. Then she started having memory issues and thought it was an early onset of dementia. Her arthritis in her legs and hips got so severe, she found it difficult to stand during her lectures and started sitting in the front of the class. Her memory issues got worse, and she found herself writing little notes to herself all day not to forget things. Her kids were startled one night when she mentioned wanting to see a movie that they had recently watched with her. She also developed dry painful eyes, dry mouth that woke her up, and her scalp became constantly itchy, to the point that she spent over $5000 on shampoos and creams for her scalp, but none of them worked. She said this symptom was extremely difficult to deal with, there was just no relief.

She went to the doctor and was eventually diagnosed with Lupus and Sjogren's and her doctors recommended she take steroids and Hydroxychloroquine but she refused to do so, afraid of side effects. She wanted a more natural way to treat her illness.

Her daughter was an ethical vegan, who ate that way because of her love for animals, and Emily found herself eating mostly vegan food because of her kids who were aged 5, 7, 16, and 18 at the time. She admitted she loved eating Tofurkey (soy products processed to taste like meat) and "a ton of Veganaise", a vegan mayonnaise that is primarily made with oil. She also occasionally ate fish, which of course was not vegan. She read Goodbye Lupus and realized her diet was inflammatory. She started drinking more water, buying pressed juices from the store, and eating some flax seeds, but found herself struggling to motivate herself, calling herself "lazy". She bought a Vitamix blender and made an appointment with me to help change her diet. After a week of trying to do it on her own, she decided to do my 4 Week Rapid Recovery Program with me.

We addressed her fears about not sticking with it, planned how to get in all of her healing foods in the most convenient way possible while working at the college. We checked in daily. During Rapid Recovery, clients eat the strictest form of my protocol that focuses on the healing properties of greens omega 3s and water. Emily found it easiest to use green smoothies, to get in all her greens, omega-3s, and a lot of her water, then drank the rest of the water all day long.

Emily was getting about a pound of greens a day.

At the 2 week mark she said she could feel "this is saving my life." She felt energized and her mind was clear. Her memory was working again! She no longer struggled to get her water in, now she was thirsty for it. Her joints were much butter, although she still had some muscle pain. Of note, her joints felt worse the first week as she got through the detox phase, and then dramatically better in the second week. This is common that during the first week people can feel more symptomatic, tired, or even flu-like symptoms, but if they stick with it one hundred percent, they emerge feeling dramatically better in the second week

Even though she was supposed to check in every day with her daily log of her foods and activities and text me any time she needed support, after our 2 week check-in call, I stopped hearing from her. I reached out to her and she told me that she was "already better and didn't want to bother me anymore! All of her symptoms had disappeared; the joint pain, the gut problems, the dry eyes and dry mouth, even the "Carpal Tunnel" and the itchy scalp! She was so amazed and grateful, she didn't want to use up my time when she didn't need me, even though it was part of her program!

Here is Emily's summary of what happened:

> "My name is Emily Horowitz, I am 46 years old. About a year and a half ago I was first diagnosed with lupus and then Sjogren's syndrome,

I had an itchy scalp, my skin was itchy, my feet were itchy, I thought I had Carpal Tunnel Syndrome, my wrists hurt all the time. I wore braces (on my wrists) and I couldn't even text. I was exhausted all the time. I had brain fog all the time. I actually started to think I had like early-onset Alzheimer's.

I would teach and my ankles would hurt so much that I started sitting down when I would lecture to a class, I was buying vitamins, I was doing everything and nothing was helping. Dr. Goldner's nutrition plan, I cannot emphasize how much it changed my life, Immediately the itching stopped. I don't have to wear braces on my wrist, I can type, I apparently don't have Carpal Tunnel Syndrome. I don't have any ankle pain, I don't have any knee pain, I had one doctor I consulted said that I had a labral tear in my hip and one option was hip surgery, I don't have any pain in my hip, I can walk everywhere, I can play with my kids.

I remember things; I don't have to write everything down. I can type, I can text. I don't take any painkillers anymore. I've had stomach problems for years and years, they're completely gone, my stomach is perfect. I can stand up in front of my class. I have energy.

It's transformed every aspect of my life and the way I feel and I hope that everybody who's suffering from any kind of autoimmune or other disorder has the opportunity to try this, I mean it will save lives."

Chapter 31
Case Study #6: Rachel's Story

Reversing Lupus & Sjogren's During Pregnancy

Rachel had lupus and Sjogren's disease when she came to me. She was also 32 weeks pregnant at the time. She had one healthy baby previously, her daughter was 3 years old at the time. After that successful pregnancy, she had a miscarriage before this pregnancy. She ended up in the hospital after both the successful pregnancy and the miscarriage because her lupus was so severe after each pregnancy. That's a common problem. In fact, many women are first diagnosed with Lupus after their first pregnancy. Rachel was diagnosed a year after the birth of her first child, although she says she realized afterwards she had been symptomatic for 6 years prior to her diagnosis.

She had many symptoms of both Sjogren's and Lupus; dry mouth and dry eyes (Sjogren's) to joint pain and the butterfly-shaped red rash known as a malar rash on her cheeks, classic for Lupus. Before being diagnosed with these illnesses, Rachel was very athletic. She loved to go to the gym and ran half-marathons regularly. She had not been able to run in years because of joint pain, and missed it very much. She also had severe back pain at the time which she thought was from the pregnancy. When she called me, she was 4 weeks and 2 days away from her scheduled C-section. We had very little time and she immediately started my 4 Week Rapid Recovery Program so we could work together every day and make sure she got better as quickly as possible.

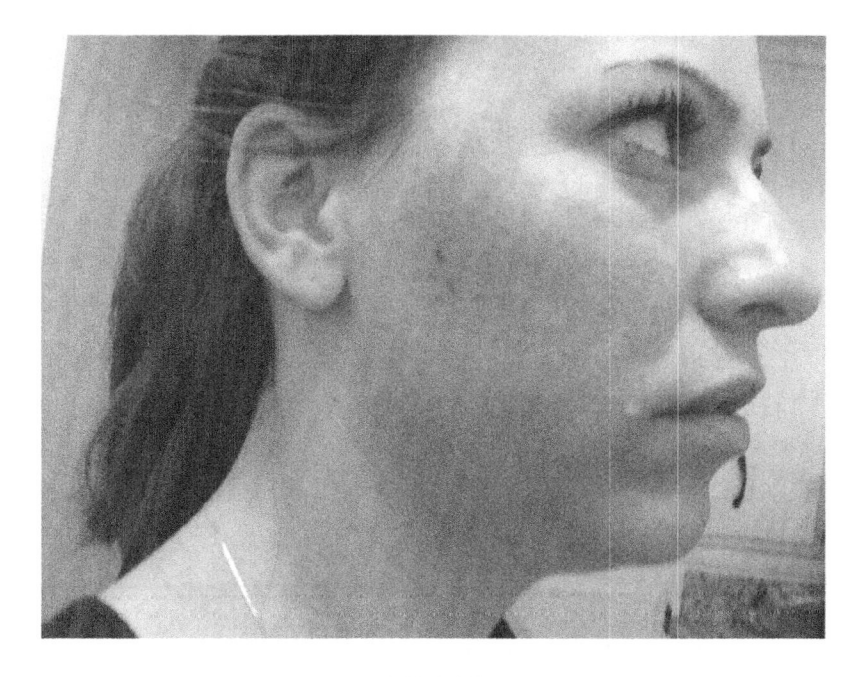

BEFORE

I occasionally get asked if it's ok to do the Rapid Recovery nutrition plan during pregnancy. The answer is a resounding, of course! What better time is there to feed yourself the healthiest foods on the planet than while you are pregnant? The same foods that reverse illness will build a healthy baby! Research supports this. For example, research has shown that pregnant women who take omega-3s have longer gestation times and children superior neurodevelopment and higher IQs.[22,23]

Even though she was scared of her illness, Rachel and her husband really wanted a sibling for their daughter and decided to try again. When I met Rachel, she was already on maternity leave, which she had to start early because she was in so much pain and exhausted all the time. She spent most of her time sleeping, which was tough since she had a young daughter that needed her. We decided to immediately start the 4 Week Rapid Recovery program. Rachel was motivated and dedicated.

She focused on drinking at least 90 ounces of green smoothie a day, eating tons of raw foods, and at least half a cup of omega-3s a day. She sent me photographs of her green smoothies and large salads, and giant raw wraps. She immediately noticed a surge in energy. Her aches and pains lifted and she realized that her back pain, that she thought was from pregnancy, had disappeared. She felt so energized she no longer needed to nap, and was up running around and playing with her daughter. By the end of the 4 weeks, she felt really good, no more dry eyes or mouth, no more pain, and her labs tests showed her Sjogren's antibodies had disappeared.

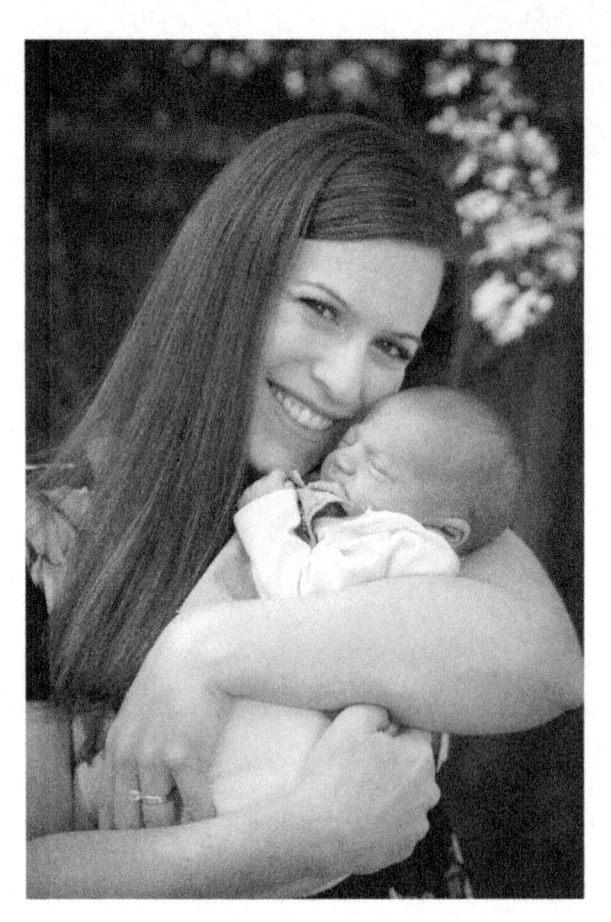

AFTER

How was she feeling after those four weeks on the protocol? I'll let Rachel tell you in her own words.

> Hi I'm Rachel, I am 34 years old and I was diagnosed with lupus three and a half years ago. I had symptoms of sun sensitivity, I couldn't be out in the sun for more than a few minutes and my skin would feel like it was on fire, I would break out in the typical lupus butterfly rash on my face sometimes within a few minutes from being outside and it was just so incredibly painful. I started becoming so fatigued, I'd come home from work and just lay on the couch, I couldn't be the mom I wanted to be for my daughter. I had so much pain in my legs I had to give up running which was a passion of mine, my husband and I decided to try for another baby I ended up with a miscarriage and after that I had a major flare up again and I was getting the butterfly rashes, I was getting fevers, I always felt like I had the flu and I was just very fatigued and my legs always hurt, just always in pain.
>
> So, my husband and I made that decision okay we're going to try again, and when I was about 8 months pregnant I started getting very scared that I was going to have this baby and be even sicker after I had him. So, when I was 8 months pregnant I heard of this book called Goodbye Lupus, so I set up an appointment with Dr. Goldner, so I completely changed the way I was eating, at 9 months pregnant I was literally four weeks from my due date it, I was so shocked. Two days into doing this I had so much energy and I felt amazing, two weeks into this when I was pregnant my shrill greens symptoms went away, my aches and pains were gone which at this point in my life I thought it was from the pregnancy but apparently not because once I started doing her protocol my pains went away, my back felt better, my legs felt better and actually one week before my due date I was running around a park teaching my almost four-year-old how to fly a kite. I gave birth to a beautiful baby boy and I had a C-section and I recovered so quickly, my baby is now five weeks old and he is amazing and I feel great and I don't have the Sun sensitivity anymore, I don't have any pains in my legs anymore, I am sitting out here in a park and I couldn't feel better.
>
> I recently just had some blood work done a week ago and a lot of this blood work markers they do to show for inflammation is negative, even my Sjogren's lab work is showing negative. So, I couldn't be more grateful for Dr. Goldner for giving me my life back, making me the

mom I want to be. My daughter comes home from school now and I play with her, I don't sit on the couch even with the lack of sleep I have with a newborn. I am running around and I am enjoying my life, I'm truly grateful for reading her book and for working with her and for continuing to work with her. I haven't felt this good in years, so thank you.

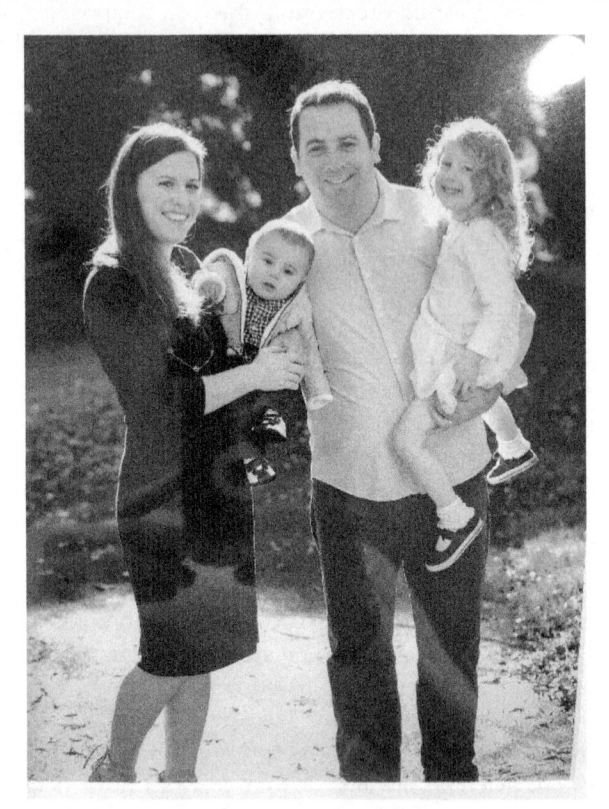

NIR BEFORE WITH DIABETES AND FATTY LIVER DISEASE

Rachel's son is now 2 years old. She is still energetic and healthy, pain and symptom free. All of her labs are completely normal, with no signs of Lupus or Sjogren's. After her labs were negative she asked her rheumatologist to taper her off her medications and he told her that was not a good idea, because even though she had zero symptoms and normal labs, the diseases are still there "because they are incurable", and therefore she should remain on medications for the rest of her life. She was very frustrated and decided to go to a new rheumatologist. The new doctor agreed with her that she does not have Lupus or Sjogren's or any autoimmune disease at all, and should come off medications. She also stated that since these diseases are incurable, it must mean that she never really had them. Rachel was stunned, and asked how she could have had all the symptoms and years of positive laboratory tests if she never had the diseases. The doctor ignored the symptoms and simply suggested it could have been lab errors. Rachel was stunned and asked her, how there could have been multiple consistent repeated lab errors, and why did she have malar rashes and joint pain and dry eyes and mouth, not to mention a miscarriage and her hospitalizations for lupus flares? The doctor had no answers for her. Rachel called me to discuss her frustrations. I sympathized that it was impressive how an intelligent educated person would create such an irrational explanation for what she was witnessing in her patient, rather than open her mind to the idea that maybe these diseases are not incurable after all, and that maybe there is a better way to treat them.

While many doctors are actively learning about how powerful nutrition is in reversing diseases, and I now get referrals from other doctors on a regular basis, there are still many doctors that are so immersed in the old ways of treating disease, where only medications and surgeries are considered viable treatments, that even when they witness people healing right in front of them, they refuse to see it. Those doctors will often offer odd, dismissive, or irrational answers, like "maybe the medications just suddenly kicked in (after 3 years)" or "I don't know what happened, but just keep doing what you're doing," or one recent doctor said, "It's a miracle ...I don't know what happened but I'm pretty sure it wasn't the food."

As a scientist, I believe it is imperative that we observe what is happening in front of us with an open mind and curiosity, not with judgment and preconceived beliefs. However, I do understand the skepticism and disbelief. I myself didn't fully realized I was truly free from lupus until my first son was born, 5 years after my symptoms had disappeared and my labs had normalized. I had just graduated from medical school at the time of my recovery, and I "knew" that lupus was incurable and I would have it for the rest of my life, so I didn't actually see what was happening within my own body, that it was really gone. I thought it was a remarkable remission, with normal lab tests and no symptoms. I kept injecting myself with blood thinners for a year after my antiphospholipid antibodies were negative, because my rheumatologist said I had to take the medicine forever because of my medical history. I finally stopped them after a year of negative labs, realizing that the risks of the medications were not justified if I had no antibodies to cause clots. After I had a healthy baby with no resurgence of lupus, I finally realized it was truly gone. As I am writing this book, it's been 14 years since my recovery from lupus, and I am still healthy and disease free, and I have helped countless others achieve the same results, so far it is a fact of life that lupus and other autoimmune diseases are reversible. I always tell my clients that if your doctor says you can't reverse autoimmune diseases that just means they have never done it or seen it, not that it isn't possible. But, having been through this awakening myself, I understand how doctors could have difficulty seeing something so unexpected and amazing. If your doctor doesn't believe it's possible, do this anyway and prove it to them.

A year after Rachel's recovery and the birth of their healthy son, Rachel's husband Nir received devastating news from his family in Israel. His mother was in the hospital, she had had a severe heart attack and was not going to survive. He was told to come to Israel to say goodbye. His mother had been sick with type II diabetes since her thirties. She had been insulin dependent since the early 1990s. According to Nir, his mother had had over 25 heart attacks since the age of 41 years old. She had had ten stents put into her heart blood vessels, and had had three bypass

surgeries. She was diagnosed with chronic heart failure 2 years prior. The doctors said her heart was "too sick to heal." Nir had just witnessed a miracle in his wife, and decided he wasn't going to Israel to say goodbye, he was going to try to save his mother. He went to the hospital armed with a Vitamix blender and started making my green smoothie recipes for her around the clock. She walked out of the hospital 5 days later. One year later, she is off of all cholesterol medicine, her legs are no longer swollen with fluid from heart failure, she has lost over 20lbs, and has normal blood sugar. She still uses a small dose of insulin, but whereas she used to take a lot of medication for her diabetes and still had an average blood sugar in the 200-300 range, she is now usually at 100 with minimal insulin. His mother recently flew to the US for the holidays and she feels great. She is energetic, she doesn't have chest pain, and she is very much alive.

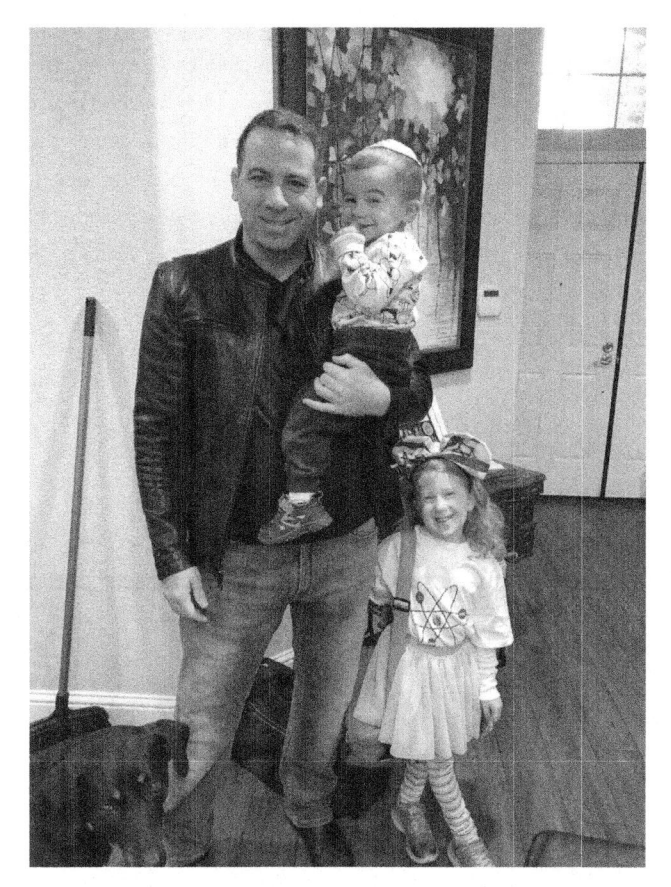

NIR HEALTHY AFTER HYPER-NOURISHMENT

After everything Nir went through with his wife and his mother, he felt grateful but also worn out from stress. While Rachel was making healthy food at home, he was eating junk food at work and he wasn't exercising. He finally made an appointment with me when he was diagnosed with type II diabetes and put on Metformin. I found out he had had non-alcoholic fatty liver disease for 15 years as well. I put him on the rapid recovery plan and taught him to do self-care for his emotional health and stress, as well as exercise. In 4 weeks, his liver enzymes were completely normal for the first time in 15 years. His 5 week labs showed normal blood sugars. He is off medication with no signs of diabetes or fatty liver, he lost weight and feels fit and healthy. He has been exercising with his wife, and they are determined to live a healthy life and raise their kids on an unprocessed plant-based vegan diet. They tell me that their daughter, who is now five years old, often tells people about Dr. G and how vegetables saved her mommy. Their little boy has been drinking green smoothies out of his bottles. Both children are healthy and strong and vibrant. Their two children have the genes for autoimmune disease, type II diabetes, fatty liver disease and heart disease, but their children will never get these diseases because their parents have changed their diets and their lifestyles to stop these diseases from progressing. We can save our kids from ever getting the illnesses that we had.

Chapter 32
Case Study #7: Meredith's* Story

A Case of Childhood Lupus

Sadly, I'm getting more and more kids with autoimmune disease as clients. At the time I was diagnosed with lupus at sixteen back in the 1990s, it was considered young. Now I'm seeing children as young as 2 with lupus. It's heartbreaking. The good news is, the protocol doesn't just work for adults. It's great for kids too. Meredith was eleven when she was diagnosed with lupus. At the time I met her and her family, she already had cardiomyopathy, an enlarged heart, and myocarditis, and infection of the heart, her kidneys were failing from lupus nephritis, and she had protein in her urine, and she also had a rash on her face. She'd had a seizure in the hospital that led to a code blue, she stopped breathing and they had to resuscitate her. I can't imagine what her mother and her father were going through watching their child being brought back to life again on tubes and machines, I talked to her distraught mother and said we can absolutely help her get her health back.

We put Meredith on the children's version of the protocol. For her size, it ended up being about half the amount as what I recommend for adults. She drank half of a blender of green smoothie a day with about 6 packed cups of leafy greens, which was about one-half to three-quarters of a pound of greens a day. In addition, we focused on finger foods like broccoli, cauliflower, and guacamole. She drank half a gallon of water a day. Within two weeks, her parents noticed remarkable results. 2 and a half weeks after our first call, her mother texted me:

> "Dr. Goldner quick update on Meredith she's gotten off two medications since our chat and her labs are trending well, her nephrologist said she no longer suffers from proteinuria."

After only two and a half weeks, her kidneys recovered.

A couple months later I received another text message from her very happy mother:

> "Another update we just had a cardiology appointment last week her heart is completely back to normal, no more fluid around her heart."

When I checked in with them a year later, mom texted me:

> "She's been doing martial arts three times a week, 1 hour each since May. She really kicks butt!! :) This is the same girl who suffered from myocarditis less than a year ago. She's a member of the student council in her school. She plays the piano and the viola. She wants to be a nephrologist when she grows up. :) Oh, and she's an honorable student, straight A's the entire year!!!"

At the time I last spoke with them Meredith was being tapered off of her medications. Meredith went from the ICU with failing organs, to the top of her class, physically active, playing music, and planning her future, Meredith is thriving.

People often ask me, "I'm doing this for me but my kids are healthy do I really need to put them on this diet?" Or they will ask, "my kids are sick, is this going to give them enough nutrition?" My answer is that if your kids are healthy, this is for them. Putting children on an unprocessed plant-based diet high in raw foods and omega-3s will give them the best possible chance of staying healthy and avoiding diseases in the future. If your kids are unhealthy, this is also for them. As you can see from Meredith's case, this protocol can quickly reverse devastating illnesses and help sick children regain their health. Why not give our children the very best food on the planet? You need to realize that your children have your genes for illness, and by eating this way you can prevent them from ever going through what you're going through right now or worse, and what better gift is there as a parent to give your child than health.

*Name changed to protect identity

Chapter 33
Case Study #8: Sarah Runco's Story

Reversing Chronic Pain, Obesity, & Cervical Dysplasia

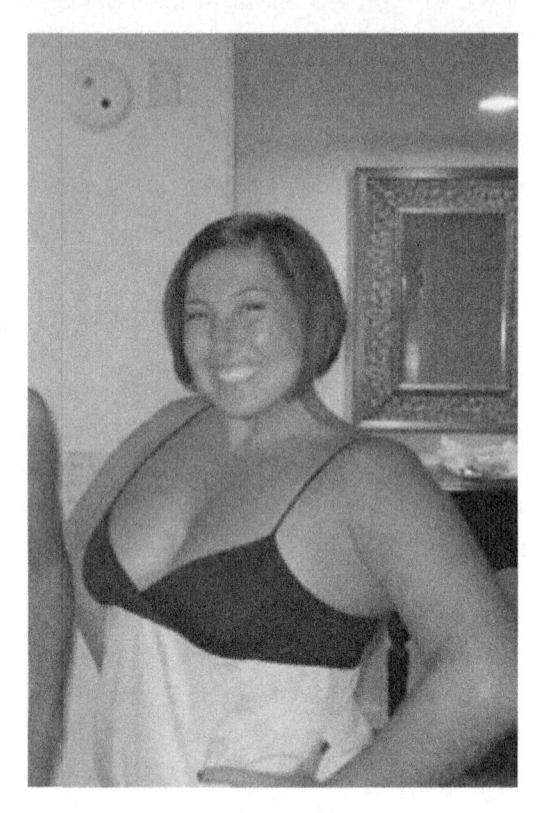

SARAH BEFORE

When I first met Sarah, she was 29 years old and suffered from chronic pain for over ten years. She didn't have an autoimmune disease diagnosis, but still had chronic inflammation. I share her case to demonstrate that you don't need an official diagnosis to benefit from the protocol. Many people are sick for five to ten years before they meet the criteria for a diagnosis of autoimmune disease. When I met Sarah, she was seeing seven doctors and on nine different medications to help her inflammation and chronic pain. She had had multiple joint surgeries, but nothing got rid of the pain. Some doctors accused her of drug-seeking because of her constant complaints of pain.

She also had chronic bladder inflammation and cervical dysplasia, pre-cancerous cells on her cervix, caused by HPV. She had had multiple surgeries to remove these pre-cancerous cells but they kept growing back. The biopsy results from her last surgery showed that there were still cells in the margin, so they hadn't gotten it all. She worried she would end up with cervical cancer.

When I met her, her favorite foods were frozen packaged foods like Lean Cuisine, chips, crackers, and packaged ramen. She also ate a lot of lunch meats or she'd have a meal of just cheese and crackers, or crackers and lunch meats and cheese. Also, lots of frozen foods. A lot of folks out there are living on processed foods and dairy products and meat and she was one of them.

I'm going to let Sarah tell her story because she's really good at sharing not only what it's like to feel better, but what it feels like to be hyper-nourished.

My name is Sarah... I was suffering from chronic pain for over ten years. I was 203 pounds, I was under the care of seven doctors, on nine medications, I had multiple surgeries on joints and I was struggling big-time. I was so discouraged. Fast forward, with Dr. G's guidance I have been pain free, I have had zero flare-ups, I have gone to zero doctor's appointments and I have not been on any pain medication.

I am so thrilled, I am a hundred and forty-seven pounds which is just a side effect of everything. I never did this to lose weight but boy is that a perk.

To have these nutrients and to feel the energy after being so lethargic and so fatigued and so drained I could not be more grateful. Thank you Dr. G. I could not do this without you. You have given me the true gift of health and I can't wait to continue this journey on healing, I can't wait to inspire others like you inspire me every day, you are Wonder Woman and I am so grateful.

Now, Sarah actually had an unexpected side effect. I knew this nutrition plan would benefit her pain and inflammation, but it did more than that. One day she sent me a video message after getting her pap smear results from her Ob-Gyn. This is what she said:

> "I just got a call from my OBGYN to tell me that my PAP was normal. I haven't had a normal PAP since 2009. Not only do I not have any precancerous cells, my HPV came back negative which means I'm no longer a high-risk patient because I don't have a chance of getting those pre-cancer cells again (crying). Thank you doctor.

What I have found over the years is that people can heal more than I ever dreamed was possible. Being trained as a western medical doctor, I learned most conditions were permanent and chronic. HPV is considered a permanent infection, yet Sarah has continued to have normal pa smears and be HPV negative for almost 2 years now. Her results are so astonishing, her gynecologist and her uro-oncologist are coming to my next online webinar classes in disease reversal! Her gynecologist started my smoothies and her chronic migraines went away!

We are taught that most serious diseases don't ever go away, all we can do is use medications or surgeries to treat the symptoms. It turns out that is only true when we stick to medications for treatment rather than lifestyle changes to treat the actual causes of the diseases and give the body what it needs to repair itself.

What I've been seeing over and over again over the years, is that this program works for whatever issue you have. The reason is that we're just supplying the cells with what they use for healing and cell repair, so your body will use these nutrients as it needs to for repair and healing. When you think about it that way, it makes sense that it can help eliminate a virus, it can help with heart disease, it can help with neuropathies, just as it helps with autoimmune disease. We're not catering to certain conditions. As you continue to nourish yourself, your body gets healthier and healthier. For people who are no longer sick with chronic illness, they notice that they rarely ever get colds or the flu, and if they do it's gone in a day or 2 rather than a week or 2. They look and feel younger as their skin is nourished and they are energized and vibrant.

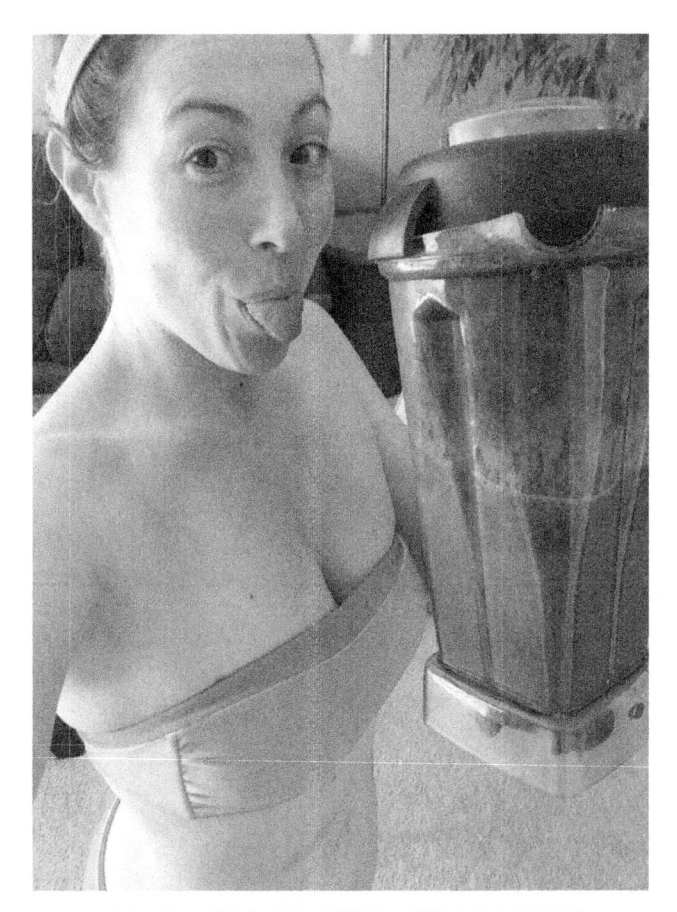

SARAH AFTER, HEALTHY AND PAIN FREE

Chapter 34
Case Study #9: Mary's Story

Reversing End Stage Kidney Failure from Lupus Nephritis

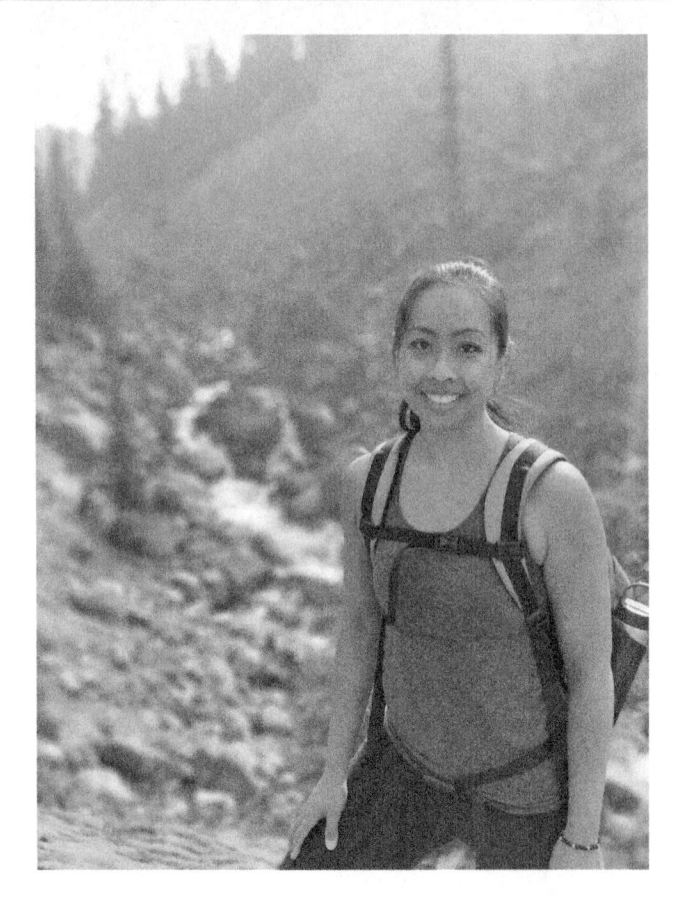

SIX MONTHS AFTER THE PROTOCOL AND ONE MONTH BEFORE GETTING MARRIED. WE HIKED FOR 9 HOURS.

Mary was diagnosed with lupus at age fifteen. When she came to me in her 20s, she only had an estimated 14% of kidney function left. Because of this, she was on the kidney transplant list and her doctors told her there was nothing more they could do, she had to get a kidney transplant.

She had been taking her meds religiously from 15 years old, she did everything her doctors told her to do, and yet she got sicker and sicker, and her kidneys continued to fail until she ended up on the transplant list while only in her twenties. She was desperate to find anything that could help her. She ended up attending online classes I taught on disease reversal and asked her doctor about doing my 6 Week Rapid Recovery Group. They told her it wouldn't help but it probably wouldn't hurt. She didn't see a reason not to at least try.

Before the protocol, she had swollen joints and slept all the time. She said she actually taught her dogs to sleep all day because she didn't have the energy to walk them. She had a loving fiancée who wanted to marry her and take care of her, but she worried for their future. She also felt like she was missing out on taking care of her little nephew. She loves him dearly, but didn't have the energy to play with him.

When Mary entered the group, she was focused and determined. I had her do the kidney failure version of the protocol using low potassium vegetables and fruits, and chia instead of flax. We had her nephrologist monitor her electrolytes and GFR every week to make sure she didn't become hyperkalemic (high blood level of potassium) or hyponatremic (low blood sodium levels) which can happen with very low kidney function. She started at the minimums of 8 cups of leafy greens, ½ cup of chia, and 96 ounces of water a day. Then she started pushing harder with my coaching and support and by the end of the 6 weeks she was drinking 2 full blenders of smoothies a day! She went from laying on the couch all day, to working out in the gym. Her pains went away, her energy was through the roof, and her labs showed her kidney function was going up every single week.

How much did she heal during the six-week rapid recovery session? I'll let her tell you.

> Hey everyone my name is Mary and I am from Richmond, DC. I was diagnosed with lupus nephritis when I was 15. I just remember being

sick all the time, I missed a lot of school work, I was achy, I was painful, I had a slight fever every day. I missed a lot of class. By January of 2017 my kidney function went down to 14% and by then I already did all the paperwork for the kidney transplant because my doctor told me it's going to happen soon and that I would need dialysis really soon. In February of 2017, Tony and I were listening to Dr. G's webinar and she was talking about starting the first group healing program and I was at the point where I was like, what do we have to lose?

After a week, I got my labs and it went up to 17% the first week! After that, every week my kidney function just has continued to increase either one, two or three percent. My last bloodwork I was at 27%! I am no longer at stage five kidney failure so that is amazing. I no longer have to take any hypertension medication; my blood pressure was so low that my doctor said stop all your medications. I was actually on two different hypertension medications at that time. They decreased my Plaquenil to three times a week and the other medications are just vitamins and it was all thanks to the healing program because it really works. (See Next Page for Lab Photo)

So, it's been about six months since I started the healing program, I have so much energy I can run around and keep up with my four and a half year-old nephew and he is full of energy. Because of the healing program I am able to become the aunt that I want to be and that he deserves. Before, I would teach my dogs how to nap because I was so tired and the three of us would just nap all day, but now we go on long walks every day after work. One thing I am looking forward to is growing old with my husband and traveling and just spending time with each other, so thank you Dr. G because without you I would not have been enjoying my life now.

I recently just saw Mary in person for the first time. She showed up at an event I was teaching in Costa Mesa. We shared lots of hugs. I'm excited to see her doing so well. It's been 2 years since she participated in the 6 Week Rapid Recovery Group and she has not needed a kidney transplant or dialysis. Mary's kidney function was down to 14% when I met her. When we got rid of all the inflammation, her function went up to 27% and plateaued there. Since she no longer has inflammation, the remaining issues are likely from sclerosis or scarring from having lupus nephritis for so long. Even if she can't regain more function than that, she is still in a very good place, because you can live with 27% kidney function and still live a normal, active life. Mary has stayed away from animal products, but occasionally will eat processed vegan foods or cooked foods, and finds that causes her kidney function to go down. People with end-stage kidney failure need to keep up the hyper-nourishment. Mary needs to continue to eat raw foods, because it allows her to live a vibrant, amazing life.

Chapter 35
Case Study #10: Stacey's* Story

Lupus & Sjogren's In Six Weeks

Stacey was living with Sjogren's and lupus. At the time that I met her, she had only been diagnosed a year ago, but her symptoms caused her a lot of pain and loss of quality of life. She was in constant pain with her joints. She also suffered from pleurisy, inflamed lungs which made it hard to breathe without terrible pain. The pleurisy was so painful and severe she ended up hospitalized for two weeks for each episode before she felt well enough to go home. Even on medications, she continued to suffer from pain and fatigue. When she contacted me, she had just gotten home from being treated at the ICU and was living with her parents.

Her dream was to be a lawyer and she had just quit law school, believing she had to give up that dream because of her health. She couldn't even hold a job because she was so disabled by her illness. When she joined the 6 Week Rapid Recovery Group, she was mostly home and in bed or on the couch, in pain and exhausted.

After only 20 days in the group, she got her first laboratory blood tests done. She was shocked to see that many of her Lupus markers like her CRP, ESR, hemoglobin, and C3 were already normal. Her rheumatologist started tapering medicine at that time. Her pain subsided and her energy levels were high. Her sleep quality was better than it ever was before. By the end of the 6 weeks, she started working and was feeling healthy. She decided to stay for another round of the group to take her health to an even greater level. She continued to hyper-nourish, and used her newfound energy to start exercising. By the end of the second round she was running for exercise. She had also re-enrolled in law school, ready to go after her dreams without the fear of Lupus or Sjogren's holding her back again. She is off medications, exercises twice a day, and is completing her law degree. She is also active on Instagram showing off her healthy food and lifestyle to inspire others to take back their health and their dreams, the way she did.

* Name was changed to protect identity.

Chapter 36
Case Study #11: Karen's Story

Primary Sjogren's In Six Weeks

Karen suffered from Sjogren's disease and antiphospholipid antibody, which causes blood clots. Other symptoms include severe dry mouth and eyes, itchy scalp, and 'burned tongue.' Burned tongue is a symptom of Sjogren's where nerve inflammation in the tongue makes it feel like it is burning. Karen found it difficult to eat or enjoy food because of this symptom.

Karen's doctor was very excited that she was joining my 6 Week Rapid Recovery Group, and decided to take lab tests before and after the program to see how much progress he could see on paper after 6 weeks. Karen was excited to have all of her symptoms disappear in the 6 weeks. She discusses her physical progress and her lab findings below.

> My name is Karen, I'm 65 and I was diagnosed a year and a half ago with Sjogren's syndrome, primary Sjogren's syndrome and I also had a diagnosis of antiphospholipid syndrome. I had the classic Sjogren's syndromes of dry eye, dry mouth but I also had burning itching feeling on my scalp that never went away. I had burned tongue syndrome 24/7 and I also had some neuropathy beginning in my toes. And so, when I found Dr. G I was ecstatic. Sometime between the second week and the sixth week of the healing program, the itching burning feeling on my scalp was gone. The burned tongue syndrome, one day I realized my tongue felt normal there was no problem there. The numbness in my toes resolved, all gone and they've stayed resolved. I have no problems during the day, plenty of saliva, plenty of tears. As far as the blood work what we found at the end of that six weeks was that the inflammation markers in my blood were back to normal no problems.
>
> My heart and liver functions were great, the blood count, white blood counts and red blood counts, completely normal. The Sjogren's antibodies are still there but it's at a low manageable level. The nutrient levels are fantastic and my liver and my kidney functions are all

normal. And the extra added thing about the cardiac testing is that my heart is fine, there are no blockages and in the vascular scans, when I said to my doctor, "so I have no blockages?" She said, "nowhere even close, you're great."

The antiphospholipid syndrome has resolved, it's not there in my blood now! What can I say? This program works. I have been given a very powerful tool in hyper-nutrition to take care of myself for the rest of my life. So, I have to say to Dr. G thank you so much, you have made such an impact and difference in my life with your hyper-nutrition program, I recommend it to everyone .

Chapter 37
Case Study #12: Mabel's Story

Rheumatoid Arthritis, Sjogren's & Graves' Disease In Six Weeks

Mabel was diagnosed with rheumatoid arthritis, Sjogren's and Graves' disease. She was first diagnosed with autoimmune disease at only 15 years old, diagnosed with Graves' (hyper-thyroid) and dry eyes. In her twenties, her lacrimal glands in her eyes (which secrete tears) started growing. They deformed her upper eyelids. In spite of the enlarged glands, her eyes remained very dry. She had multiple surgeries on them but they kept growing back. Doctors diagnosed her with Sjogren's-like syndrome at that time. Her salivary gland was also enlarged as well.

In spite of having medical issues her whole life, she became a medical doctor, got married and had a family. The symptoms became worse over time, and when she joined my 6 Week Rapid Recovery Group at age 38, she was struggling with chronic joint pain that was so bad she couldn't sleep because of the pain. She had "horrible anxiety" about her health and being able to be a mother to her children. She used Systane for eye dryness but still suffered with severe dry eyes. She was also recently diagnosed with a 5cm mass on her right ovary and was told she needed surgery.

After the 6 Week Rapid Recovery Group, Mabel found that she no longer needed any eye drops at all. Her glands in her eyes stopped growing and she no longer needed surgery to contain them. After over 20 years of autoimmune disease, her ANA (an autoimmune marker) was negative. As a doctor, she was stunned! Also, the 5cm mass on her ovary simply disappeared.

Here's what she had to say about her experience:

> My name is Mabel* and I'm a doctor right now. I'm living in Florida. When I was 15, I was diagnosed with Graves's syndrome, Sjogren's-like syndrome and rheumatoid arthritis. I've been living with pain all my life. I had some ovary issues, a large tumor on my right ovary. I started with a group of beautiful women who are feeling the same way

as I was. It was amazing. I just couldn't believe it was so fast, I couldn't believe what I was seeing, I'm healing.

My anti-nuclear antibodies were negative and my inflammatory markers were very low. I did an ultrasound for my ovary; the mass was 5 centimeters and now there's nothing there! I'm so thankful for everything that's happened and for everything that Dr. Goldner has taught me, and for a very good group of friends that has been so supportive, thank you Dr. Goldner for everything. This is the best thing that has ever happened to me.

After a lifetime of autoimmune disease, Mabel finally is empowered to care for herself. She has hope and a path to a better healthier life.

* Name was changed to protect identity

Chapter 38
Case Study #13: Arthiraani Ramalingam's Story

Hashimoto's Disease In Six Weeks

Now Arthi is someone with hypothyroid disease. Hashimoto's is one of the most common autoimmune diseases out there and I see a lot of clients with it. One of the problems in Western medicine is that with Hashimoto's, all doctors do is give you back your thyroid hormone after the autoimmune disease kills your thyroid. But they do nothing to get rid of the autoimmune disease, so the process continues. Even with thyroid hormone replacement, people often feel tired, experience brain fog, and have difficulty losing weight. They also develop arthritis from continued inflammation from the untreated autoimmune disease underlying the thyroid disease.

Arthi was struggling with those exact issues: she was overweight and couldn't get her weight to budge, she felt sluggish and tired, and arthritic. When Arthi first joined the group her pain was a three out of ten, her energy was low, and her mood was only a 5 out of 10. A lot of people with Hashimoto's battle depression as well.

6 weeks later, she ranked her pain as zero, energy was high, mood was 10 out of 10! She was exercising, and she was fitting into the clothing size she hadn't been since high school! So, she loved this program, she was showing us pictures of herself and her skin was glowing and feeling great. During the group she would update us saying things like, "I'm so proud of my skin health!" "I do push-ups like a pro and my strength while exercising is phenomenal given how saggy I would feel before!" "My blouse fit me from eight years ago!".

She has gone on to be what I call a health missionary, where she tells everyone she can about how beneficial this program is for hypothyroid. I sometimes wonder if she gets google alerts to let her know when someone posts about hypothyroid, because she shows up so quickly to comment, encourage and tag me on social media! Recently, I got tagged with "Dr. Goldner starting another group and you should join that group. I just finished revealing and it was nothing short of miraculous".

If you've got hypothyroid disease, you need to hyper-nourish yourself to get your body healthy again. It will eliminate the chronic inflammation that is triggering the disease, and alleviate the low energy and the brain fog and give you a fast metabolism. People often ask me, can I get off my thyroid medicine? That depends if you have an active thyroid. After years of inflammation damaging the gland, it can become scarred and no longer active, just like the kidney that become scarred and sclerotic over time. The only way we know how much active thyroid you have is after you have been committed to the program and reach a plateau. If your thyroid is inflamed then getting the inflammation down with this program should help you get function back.

But if your thyroids already scarred over or essentially dead, this will get rid of all the other symptoms that the autoimmune disease is causing and then you just continue to replace the thyroid hormone. At least it's just the hormone that you've lost that you're replacing and not a more severe immunosuppressant medication that people typically take for autoimmune.

For some folks I have seen, they completely came off their thyroid replacement hormone and had normal function again. For many others, they are able to lower their thyroid replacement hormone as some of the thyroid heals but other parts can no longer function. In recent groups, I had 2 members with hypothyroid who suddenly got symptoms of hyper-thyroid (shaking, loose stool, anxiety from too much thyroid hormone) halfway through the group because their thyroid function had gone up, and now their thyroid replacement medication was causing them to have too much thyroid hormone! They lowered their medications with their prescribing doctors assistance and felt much better.

People also ask about cruciferous vegetables with hypothyroid because you often hear that they hurt thyroid function or cause goiters. I have never had a client grow a goiter from eating cruciferous vegetables, while I have seen many get their thyroid function back. Cruciferous vegetables are the most nutrient-dense vegetables you can get at the supermarket, and they are important for healing. Just make sure you also have iodine intake. You don't need a lot of iodine though. The Recommended Daily Allowance (RDA) is only 150 micrograms a day. For perspective, one teaspoon of iodized salt contains approximately 250 micrograms of iodine. Having some dulse seaweed once or twice a week has been found to deliver an enormous wallop of iodine (72 micrograms of iodine in only one gram of dulse). You can also use iodized salt or an occasional iodine supplement, but you don't want to go over the recommended amounts, because that has the potential to worsen issues with your thyroid as well.

Chapter 39
Case Study #14: Dawn Ingram's Story

Rheumatoid Arthritis In Six Weeks

Dawn has had rheumatoid arthritis for many years to the point that she has joint deformities. People with Rheumatoid arthritis can get something called ulnar deviation, where all of their fingers start to bend towards their pinky finger and the joint actually disfigures and gets stuck that way. It's painful, all the muscles are constantly pulled to the side, and they lose the function of their fingers. Dawn had pretty severe ulnar deviation and pain in her fingers. She couldn't brush her hair or even feed herself without intense pain. She also had severe pain and limited mobility in her arms and shoulders and legs. She struggled just to get out of bed and would hold onto the railing and limp slowly down the steps in the morning. Her legs and feet were painfully swollen. She felt depressed and isolated.

Something that I love about Dawn is that, in spite of years of suffering, she never stopped believing in her heart there was a path to healing besides medication. The medications made her feel terrible, so she didn't take them and went instead to functional medicine doctors and naturopaths but they didn't have answers for her. She got to the point that she was stuck in bed. She started making videos of herself, tracking her illness and her symptoms, hoping one day they would be the "before" videos once she found a way to heal. It was also her form of therapy for herself.

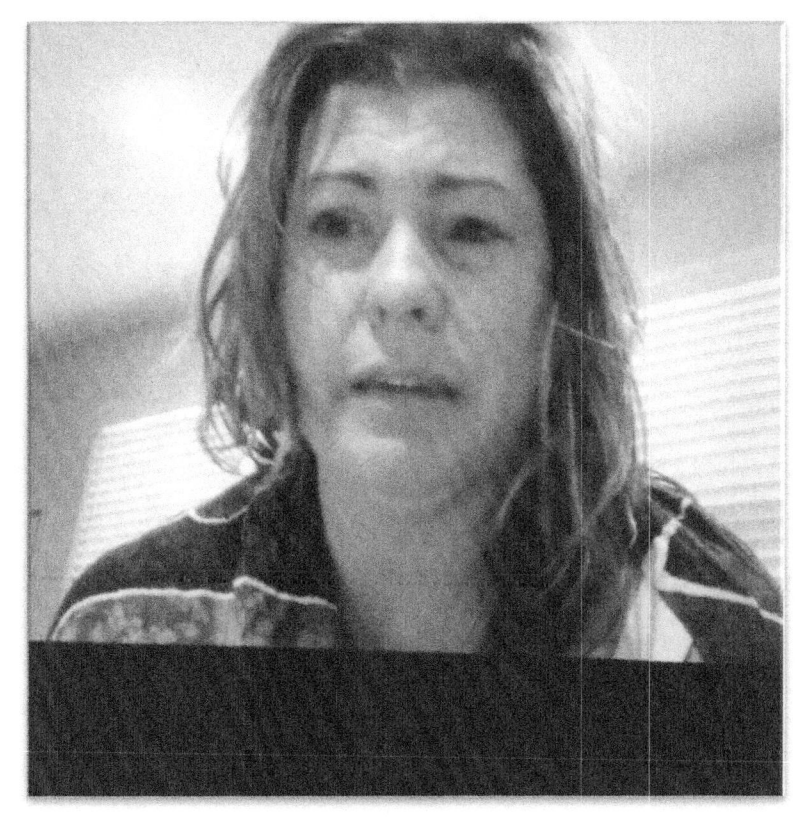

BEFORE

She started trying all different kinds of nutrition plans, she tried everything she could find through google, and nothing worked at all until she found my program and started trying to hyper-nourish herself. She found my book she found my protocol and for the first time in her life she started to feel better. Excited by her first ever breakthrough, she joined my 6 Week Rapid Recovery Group, and her life has transformed.

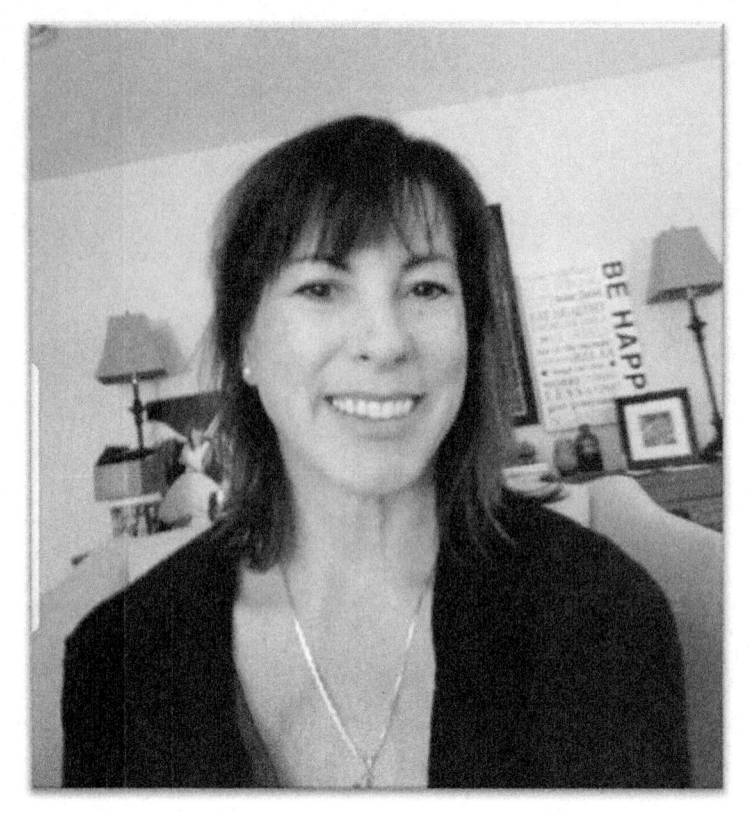

AFTER

My husband runs the Rapid Recovery Group with me which is an enormous benefit to members. Not only did he create the original version of this protocol that healed me, he's brilliant at understanding and teaching cellular biology and metabolism. He also has a background in personal training and has dozens of certifications. He currently is a motivational speaker who teaches huge audiences the mindset for success, helping entrepreneurs get over the mental barriers that keep them from achieving their dreams. That combination of skills has made him an incredible asset to the group.

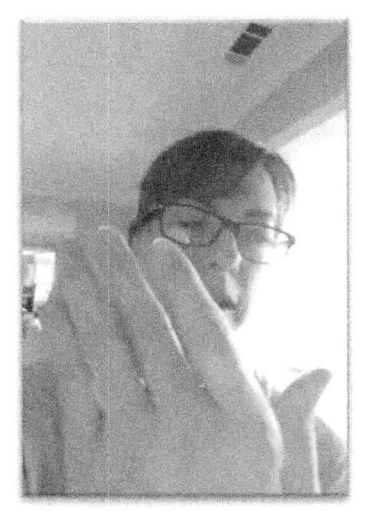

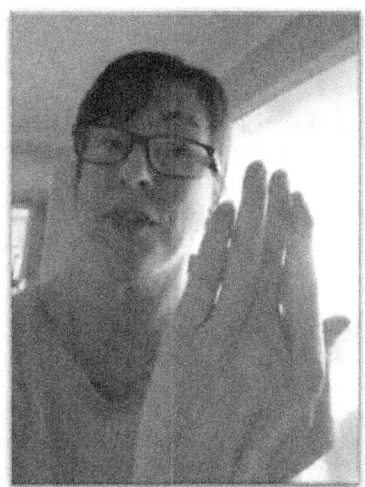

FINGERS BEFORE   FINGERS AFTER

After only 3 weeks in the Rapid Recovery Group, Dawn posted a video of her moving her fingers back to the midline, something she hadn't been able to do in years. She was excited by her increased mobility and wanted to optimize her ability to use her hands again. To do this, Dawn hired Thomas to help her with physical therapy techniques to strengthen her hands while she was hypernourishing in the group. He had her exercise her fingers to build strength multiple times a day.

By the end of the group, Dawn was literally dancing in her home with happiness. She could take the steps one at a time, she had full range of motion in her shoulders, hips, and knees, and felt energetic and happy. Dawn sent me a video testimonial to share showing her amazing progress, and I wish you could see it here. I will share what she said below, but I encourage you to look for Dawn on my website or YouTube page and see for yourself!

> Hey! this is Dawn from Savannah. I just finished the rapid healing group. I had been really, really sick and I had joint pain, neuropathy, edema, connective tissues, ringing in the ears, hair loss, stuck in bed most of the time, chronic fatigue. To get out of the bed it would probably take me about three minutes, and then another five that if I wanted to go from here to just where that door is (about 6 feet away),

it probably would have taken me like five minutes to shuffle there. And it would have been excruciating.

I had just excruciating pain that would happen in the shoulders, it's like an ice pick through here (points to shoulders) and maybe my arms could move like this (shrugs shoulders slightly).

So, I can now, I can do this way (raises arms straight over her head), can do this way (puts her arms straight out to the sides), over my head.

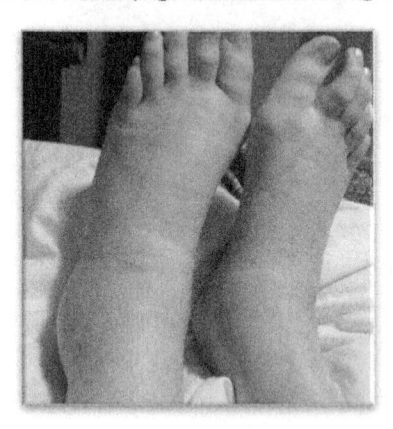

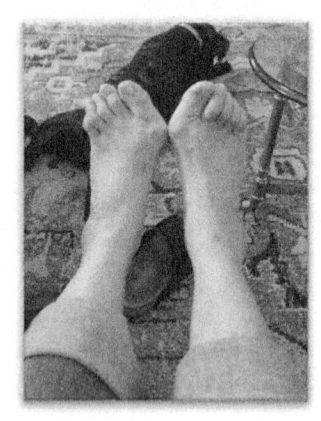

FEET BEFORE FEET AFTER

I can brush my hair, brush my teeth feed myself. Before, I would try to go to dinner with somebody, I would need to order something that I don't have to cut, because I can't actually hold my silverware and cut food. I can barely hold it to get it to my mouth. I can feed myself now!

One of my party tricks is the fact that you see that with my hand the fingers go that way (all fingers bent towards the pinky side), but if I focus I can now move them back to the left (straightens fingers). I can clap now, can you imagine, I couldn't imagine this before! Drumming my hands on the table! I can open my water!

I was laid up in the bed, could hardly have a sheet on me. It hurt to move, I had to keep my legs propped up. I can now easily get out of my chair and move it and I just want to show you I can walk about the room, change directions, and do things with no problem.

My Shower is a tub shower, so trying to get in the shower to pick up my leg was almost impossible. And I just want to show you now I can actually do high knees, let alone just normal stepping. That mobility just got better and better and better.

When you do the protocol, if you really commit to it, I mean that's all in, that is for real and you go hyper-nourishing all the way, that's when a lot of these other things that I couldn't really do before, really started getting better, like that I could really put a ponytail in my hair or just function.

When you're that sick, it's sad, your expectations aren't like I want to climb Kilimanjaro, you're like, I just want to get up and get dressed and not be in the bed, and now I can. So, I don't want you to think that I just kind of felt a little bad when I started.

It was the first time in my entire life that I had ever done any kind of a protocol and had success. I've been busting my tail and working and trying to do these other protocols and I'm getting sicker and sicker and I don't understand. I don't understand why nobody can tell me what's wrong with me, why can't anybody help me?

Dr. G. is amazing, she is totally there for you. If you do this 6-week group, and just as a small aside, if you are concerned about her ability to work with you through the dynamic of a Facebook group, because I actually was a little worried about it, I thought how can she really? It's gonna be chaotic and how's it gonna work? Well, she has her health to a science and she has her Facebook to a science. It's amazing, it is so well organized!

The other thing that happened though, probably on week 2, was I had walked down the stairs and didn't even realize that I actually didn't shuffle down the stairs, I walked down them! I had to go back up and do it again just to make sure it wasn't a fluke!

Doing the group, she will give you tremendous support. She is a genius, she comes from the greatest place of love, and she has got to be the most organized person I've ever known. Because to be able to manage all that so beautifully, well done Dr. G, well, well done! I applaud you, and I love you tons and tons.

She's amazing, she's still going strong, she actually can do even more. I'm so excited for her. I can't wait to see what she is able to do next, and I hope you're seeing what's possible for you.

Chapter 40
Case Study #15: Angela's Story

CREST Syndrome, Scleroderma In Six Weeks

Angela diagnosed with lupus in 2004. She actually progressed to something called CREST syndrome. CREST syndrome is a widespread connective tissue disease characterized by changes in the skin, blood vessels, skeletal muscles, and internal organs. CREST is an acronym for the clinical features that are seen in a patient with this disease, (C) - Calcinosis: calcium deposits in the connective tissues, (R) - Raynaud's phenomenon: where the hands and feet turn white and cold and then blue, in response to cold or anxiety, (E) - Esophageal dysfunction resulting in swallowing difficulty (S) - Sclerodactyly: thick and tight skin on the fingers, caused by an excess of collagen deposits within skin layers, and (T) - Telangiectasia: small red spots on the hands and face that are caused by the swelling of tiny blood vessels. She also had severe Sjogren's that caused dry mouth and eyes. She said she had not produced saliva for many years, causing painful dental problems. She also had Barrett's esophagus, a complication of long standing esophageal reflux where the lining of the esophagus starts to change to resemble the lining of the intestines, and is considered a high cancer risk. She also had Hashimoto's and arthritis and fibromyalgia. She was suffering so much. She was one of those people that just everything was breaking down, and she really, really hated what happened to her skin. Her skin on her face had become red and hardened, making her look older. She hated the way she looked. She was just really depressed by all of the different things going on with her and Angela really struggled at first in the group.

This is one of the most beautiful things about the group is that, it's okay if you struggle: nobody judges you, nobody comes down on you as long as you keep posting and letting me help you and letting everyone else support you, you will keep going.

She had amazing and rapid results. By day 16, she got her saliva back! She was in the group with another woman I will introduce you to named Joyce, and both of them started producing saliva after only 16 days in the group. It was saliva day! Angela said she was drooling because she wasn't used to having water in her mouth. She was excited about her results and motivated.

Then, halfway through the group, something happened where she started to get depressed, and she started eating candy bars and unhealthy off-protocol foods. She was depressed and frustrated, but she kept posting and let us give her the support she needed to get back on track. It wasn't just me, but the entire group gave her love and encouragement to get back on track. I helped her process what happened. We worked on her triggers for poor eating like what she was thinking when she decided to eat off plan, and what were the thoughts and beliefs that led her to feel depressed. We also addressed her fears about recovery. As I taught you in earlier chapters, it can be scary to suddenly feel healthy after years of being sick. People sometimes fear what their life will be like, and if there will be new expectations for them when they are well. I helped her face her fears and get back on it and she came back with renewed commitment and determination. She completed the program and she did great. She wants you to know that even if you struggle, you don't have to be perfect, but you just have to pick up and keep going. So, I'm going to let her tell her story. If you get a chance to watch the video she made on my YouTube channel or at Goodbye Lupus.com, you can see that she literally looks like she had a facelift! Her skin is soft and glowing, and her eyes sparkle with happiness. Here is what Angela had to say after the group ended.

> Hi, my name is Angela, I started this program six weeks ago with Dr. Goldner. I had pain and inflammation. I couldn't go out in the sun. I had GERD really bad, edema in my ankles. Sjogren's, Hashimoto's, CREST Syndrome, Raynaud's, scleroderma. I have been disabled since 2010, unable to work. I was just lethargic, my hair was falling out, the flares were just unbearable, the pain was unbearable. I didn't want to live, but I started the 6 Week Rapid Recovery Group. This program has I mean literally changed my life. It's the best thing, the single best thing I've ever done in my entire life. Dr. G, has so much knowledge that you can't go wrong, and being in the group environment, if I didn't go through it with the group, I would never made the six weeks. They're always there for you, 24/7. You get to talk to somebody just to say, hey, I'm struggling or hey, guess what I did today.

She goes through your journals every day and she talks to you about certain things. If you increase this, this will happen. I noticed energy the second or third day. I could just feel like jumping bean inside. I wanted to do things. It was so fast! The swelling was gone within a week and within two weeks, I started getting saliva again. My eyes are better... I have moisture in my eyes and that's so unusual. My hair stopped falling out from hypothyroidism, and I have Barrett's esophagus, I don't have GERD! I have hair, that is growing like crazy.

My skin is better, my face looks better: it's fuller, I don't have as many wrinkles as I did when I started. I couldn't be in the sun, now I can go in the sun. I can go out there in the garden.

I hated vegetables let me tell you. Your taste buds change. This changes you from the inside out. My doctors were like, it's incurable, you can't change this, this is something that you're stuck with. And thanks to Dr. G, I'm not stuck with it. Because of this group, I think that I can go back to work. I can play with my grandchildren. I'm gonna be able to do all the things that somebody else had to do for me, enjoy life.

Oh, you won't get if you don't go through her group, this amazing support. It's just amazing, I can't say enough about Dr. Goldner nutrition plan and her support without that I would have stayed sick. I'm going to miss it, I mean I already miss it. I can do this thanks to you Dr. Golder. Thank you for all that you did for us. It was well worth every penny; your amazing love shows right through everything you say and do and so I highly recommend Dr. G's program. Not all the money in the world could get you, what you're getting in this, your health. You can't get this kind of help anywhere else for your health, do it for you. I am amazed, I am just amazed. Thank you Dr. G.

As you can tell from what she said, the support of the group was essential for her recovery. Many other people who have tried and failed on their own; they told me they only lasted two or three weeks maximum before giving up. The friendships and support in the group have been life- changing for many people who struggled to stick with it on their own. I have found that the love among the members of the group is often a powerful motivator in addition to the personal help I provide each member. They truly become a family during the 6 weeks they spend together, and most of them are still in touch with each other, sharing victories and inspiring each other for years to come after they graduate.

Chapter 41
Case Study #16: Genie Holleman's Story

Lupus & Antiphospholipid Antibodies In Six Weeks

Genie Holleman's was recently diagnosed with lupus when she joined my 6 Week Rapid Recovery Group at 69 years old. She had a positive ANA, anti-DSDNA and antiphospholipid antibody. Now even though her diagnosis was recent, she'd been in pain and exhausted for about five years before her diagnosis. A large number of my clients report to me that they are symptomatic for five to ten years before their labs finally show that they have autoimmune disease. They tell their doctors that they are tired and in pain, but since their labs still look okay, or are just have minimal changes, so they do not meet criteria for a diagnosis and they are sent away. Some tell me their doctors say "you don't have autoimmune yet, but you will, and when you do we will start medication," or some even get sent to the psychiatrist or put on an antidepressant, feeling unheard and misunderstood.

After a few years, the labs finally catch up with how sick they truly are and they are diagnosed. Part of them feels glad to be validated as actually being sick, and part of them is terrified of the diagnosis and the medicines used to treat them. Labs often take time to correlate with the symptoms that you feel.

That is why I always caution people not to rely on just your labs for how you feel you are doing. Just like it can take five years for your labs to confirm that you have lupus when you've been feeling like hell for five years, during recovery, people often quickly feel extraordinary; they are running, jumping, skipping, and feeling so good, even while their labs are still not all negative yet. Some of my clients have rapid changes in their labs, as you have read in previous chapters where the inflammation markers and antibodies drop like a rock in only a matter of weeks, and for other people, their symptoms improve far more rapidly than their labs. Remember Danielle, who was running 5Ks and no longer had neuropathies or photosensitivity, but it took over 6 months for her anti-DSDNA antibodies to normalize. That is why I recommend you rely on your symptoms as your primary marker for recovery, your labs will catch up when they catch up. Listen to your body; you know when you're sick, and you know when you're healing.

Genie had been sick for so long and nobody was helping her. She had lower leg edema, she had intermittent purpura, she had arthritis, she had fatigue. She also had very high stress: her daughter and her grandchildren had moved in with her. She was taking care of all of her grandkids while her daughter worked, homeschooling them. She didn't know she could do this program, because she also had to cook for her family and she was still cooking them the stuff they wanted, while trying to hyper-nourish herself. She had a lot of food cravings, as most people do at first, and she was literally making the foods she was craving. She was surrounded by cookies and soda as well, things that would tempt her immensely when she felt low.

Genie's husband relied on her to cook for him and her daughter and grandkids did too, and they were not favorable to giving up meat and dairy and processed foods. I encourage people to ask for as much support as possible while they are on the recovery plan. For example, a spouse who isn't going along with the program can usually make his or her own meals, and meals for the kids or grandkids They might not like it, but hopefully they are supportive enough to take on that role and help you. Of course, optimally, everyone will eat healthy plant-based foods and nourishing smoothies and salads, but sometimes the person doing the program is not supported by their partner and has to find a way to do it on their own.

I strongly encouraged Genie to ask her husband or daughter for help, or at least just buy healthy foods even if they are cooked, so she wouldn't be tortured by junk food while trying to overcome her own food addictions. She decided it would be too hard to make others around her change or step up, so she decided to fight through her cravings and make them the unhealthy food they wanted while also sticking with the Rapid Recovery Protocol for herself.

Genie struggled to make herself a priority. She did a wellness consultation with me online but ultimately gave up on her nutrition program because it was inconvenient and stressful to try to eat better in her home environment. Her decision that eating on plan would burden others was a symptom of her difficulty with believing she was worth it, and that she didn't need to always be pleasing to others. We worked hard in the group on her self-esteem, and fighting her constant cravings for the unhealthy food surrounding her on a daily basis.

Because of her tendency to put herself last also showed up as a reticence to do self-care. She was constantly doing things for her family, and didn't feel like she had time to take a long bath or meditate or exercise. During the 6 weeks in the group, I had to do a lot to help her understand that even with all that stress and everything else going on, she could and should still take care of emotional health. That as long as she put herself last, she would never get her health back. I often remind my group members that it was their old habits around eating and self-care that got them sick, and if they want to heal, they need to let go of old habits and embrace a new way of talking to themselves, treating themselves, and feeding themselves. That was really transformative for her. She let go of the belief that taking care of herself meant she was not taking care of her family, and realized that taking great care of yourself is how you take care of your family. Her emotional and physical transformation was incredible. I am so proud of Genie! Here is what she had to say after she finished the 6 Week Rapid Recovery Group.

> I'm Genie... I'm 70. I was diagnosed this year with late onset lupus. I did research on lupus and through doing that I found Dr. Goldner testimony. I bought her book, I read it, and I set up a Skype consult with her last year and talked to her. She was so supportive, I thought, "you know, hey I'll do this on my own." She gave me all the information I need. I bought a Vitamix, so I could make better smoothies. But you know what, it was before the holidays and I wanted to eat the foods.
>
> We have a daughter and five grandkids living with us, and that's extra going on all the time and I just didn't do it. I didn't think there was any way I could see doing something like this and much less afford it. Then it got to be after Christmas and my doctor said, you know you have lupus. So, I thought about something Dr. G had said to me in our Skype consult, when I was telling her all the reasons, I couldn't do this. She said, "why don't you think you're worth it?" And I thought, "I am worth doing this for!" Finally, I thought that, and I decided I was going to do it.

And so, I signed up. A week and a half after I started the program, I wasn't tired anymore, I wasn't waking up tired. My mood was better. The emotional healing in this group is almost as good if not as good as the nutritional healing. Even though the stress in my life hasn't changed, my ability to cope with it has. And that's just a gift.

Oh my gosh, my nails have always been thin and papery and they peeled, and I couldn't keep polish on because they peeled. I noticed in the middle of the six weeks that, hey my nails are strong and they're slowly growing out and getting rid of all the thin, peeled areas.

My skin, especially on my arms, it doesn't look old and crepey anymore. I had swelling in my feet, and I noticed about a week ago, hey you know I can put on a pair of flats and my feet don't flow out of it. And my ANA, which has been positive for five years, is negative, My Double strand DNA which has been going up, it's coming down. And I also had an antiphospholipid antibody which makes your blood want to clot and so you can have strokes. It's normal, it's really normal, and I don't have to worry about a stroke from some stupid antibody that's floating around my body, and that is such a gift.

And I just need to tell you that this program truly can reverse your body on a cellular level. It truly can reverse labs, and Dr. G is a gift. I don't know how many times she said, I am here for you and she helps you step-by-step with whatever it is you're struggling through. There is not a better gift you can give yourself than doing this 6-week group.

I tried it on my own, I was totally committed, I couldn't do it I needed her support and the support of the other ladies doing the group. So, it just it's the best thing I ever did for myself and I am worth it.

One of the most important transformations for Genie was the psychological one. If she continues to prioritize herself, she can stay well and not let lupus or other diseases creep back into her life and steal her energy, her health, or her joy again.

Chapter 42
Case Study #17: Joyce Tompkins' Story

Sjogren's, Hypothyroid, Myopathy & Peripheral Nervous System Disorder In Six Weeks

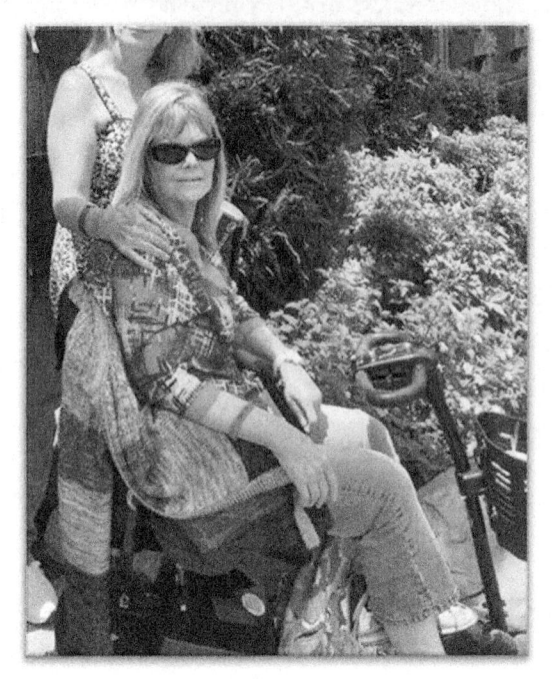

BEFORE

Joyce has had Sjogren's since 2006, as well as hypertension, Myopathy, Hypothyroidism, GERD, and a Peripheral Nervous System disorder, which caused imbalance. She also had Raynaud's disease and very limited mobility. It was very difficult for her to get around. When she joined the group, she either used a cane or a scooter to get around and her doctors told her she was going to end up full time in a wheelchair.

Her doctors insisted that there was no getting back the mobility that she had lost, it was only going to get worse. She didn't want to believe that and she joined my group. One of the first things she noticed was a dramatic increase in her energy. She thought hypothyroidism and her other conditions doomed her to feeling exhausted all the time, but she felt energetic. Suddenly, on day 16, her saliva came back after her mouth being completely dry for over 20 years. She couldn't believe it. Even more exciting, was that her pains melted away, and she started feeling stronger and more balanced.

She told me she was walking to an appointment holding her cane in her arms, not actually using it on the ground. At the end of the group she was walking around her house without any cane or scooter at all.

This is what Joyce had to say after just 6 weeks in the group doing Rapid Recovery.

> My name is Joyce Tompkins, and I was diagnosed with Sjogren's Syndrome approximately 12 years ago, thyroid disease, mixed connective tissue disease, hypothyroidism, myopathies. The Sjogren's has attacked the nerves in my limbs, making it difficult for me to get around. Eventually, I had to depend upon a cane to get around. My doctors told me that I would eventually, probably end up in a wheelchair for the rest of my life.
>
> I have had no energy to be able to go to church, to go watch our grandson play baseball, anything would wipe me out, I would need one or two naps a day. The brain fog has made me have to make a list to be able to remember things. Since I've started this six-week rapid healing group my energy level has just practically gone through the roof. Within just a few days following the protocol, I no longer needed to have a nap every day.
>
> I have been able to go watch our grandson play baseball, I no longer have to make a list. It's unbelievable, I feel like I'm alive in my body! The greatest thing is, I have saliva in my mouth now, no longer do I have dry mouth, that happened within just a couple of weeks. I've just recently had a dental cleaning and my dental hygienist was thrilled to see saliva in my mouth again and notice a dramatic improvement in my gums.
>
> I can get around pretty well without having to use the cane. I received so much encouragement and support from others within the group. It's one of the best things that I ever did for myself, I just can't thank Dr. Goldner enough for having the compassion and the drive to help

those of us that are sick. I just will be totally indebted to her for the rest of my life, my life will never be the same.

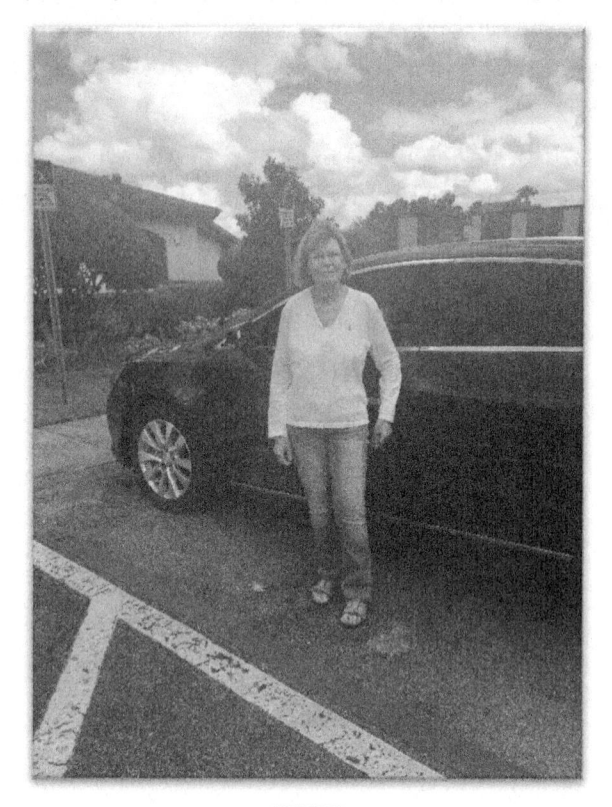

AFTER

Chapter 43
Case Study #18: Mariana Sausedo's Story

Lupus Cerebritis In Six Weeks

Mariana has had autoimmune disease since she was a child. She is someone else who always listened to her doctor, took her medication, and continued to get sick. She has had Lupus since she was 14 years old. While she had learned to live with the chronic pain and fatigue and build a life for herself living on her own and travelling with her boyfriend, she lost everything when her lupus got devastatingly worse in 2018. The lupus antibodies had crossed into her brain and she started getting daily seizures from brain lupus, or lupus cerebritis. While lupus more commonly affects the kidneys or the lungs, it can also affect the brain, where it could cause psychosis and seizures. Mary lost her independence completely, she had to move back home with her parents and it broke her heart. She also was in far worse pain and experienced a lot of hair loss.

The seizures continued to worsen and Mariana ended up in the ICU. She was having seizures every day, multiple times a day they had her on IV steroids and she couldn't stop with the seizures. When she left the hospital, her anti-double stranded DNA (anti-DSDNA) antibody (the lupus-specific antibody) was 3356 IU/ml, which was a record for that Hospital. More commonly lupus antibodies are in the 50-300 IU/ml range with active disease, the mean being 294 IU/ml.[24] When I was diagnosed with lupus at 16 years old, my anti-DSDNA antibodies was in the 2000s which they thought was extraordinarily high back then. Hers was much higher than that, and all of those antibodies were causing a lot of damage. Mariana called me from the ICU and asked if I could help her. At the time, I had a 6 Week Rapid Recovery Group starting in a week and I told her to jump into that group.

When people ask me for help, I usually lay out a lot of options. If you're not that sick you can totally take your time with this, you can start adding healing foods, you can start trying to figure it out on your own and then if it doesn't work out, you can reach out to me for an appointment or Rapid Recovery program. But if you are at the point where you have severe symptoms of autoimmune disease, you're having seizures from lupus, your kidneys are failing, you've got heart or lung disease or you just can't be in pain anymore, then I usually say join the group and let's get you better as fast as possible.

Her family didn't think joining the group as soon as she got home from the hospital was a good idea. They told her, "why not give yourself time to rest?" Thankfully, she didn't want to rest, she wanted to recover, she didn't want to wait.

After starting the group, after six weeks going right into the group from the hospital her anti-DSDNA went down to 136 IU/ml by the end of the first month on the plan. A couple weeks later, she was down to 106 IU/ml, and the last lab she had right after the group ended, her anti-DSDNA antibody level was only 84 IU/ml. There was no change in her medication, that was just the nutrition and lifestyle interventions in the group. Her seizures slowed down rapidly as well, from five to three seizures a day, to one a day, to having them only occasionally, to stopping completely by the end of the six weeks. She had never felt that healthy before in her memory. The first thing she decided to do when she was well was to go backpacking abroad, she literally got her bag and went on vacation while in the group, it was really extraordinary. She no longer gets seizures, her hair is growing, she's just feeling amazing, she took her life back.

This is what Mariana had to say in a video she made after her experience with the group.

> My name is Mariana Sausedo. I was diagnosed with lupus at the age of 14, coming up on 10 years I've had it now, but I've always had autoimmune problems being anemic to alopecia at the age of 10, shingles at the age of 12, 14 lupus, 18 RSD which is nerve damage to your foot. Fatigue to sun sensitivity, stomach issues, arthritis pain, high blood pressure, being hospitalized. Learning that "you're having seizures because lupus is attacking your brain." I got sent back home and I was either going to come home and cry and be all sad at the fact that I got sick again, or I was going to do something about it, like really do something.
>
> So, I found Dr. Goldner, I started her six-week program, and the first thing to heal was my pain. I woke up and I was pain-free. My hands didn't ache, I didn't have trigger fingers, I wasn't achy, and I've always

been achy, let me tell you that. I've always had some type of swollenness, arthritis pain, and within the next three weeks my energy was fully back. I'm on this high right now where I feel incredible, I really do. All 23 years of my life I have never been this healthy. I have always been sick, and until this program I've always thought I wasn't ever really good at anything; what I was good at was being sick. I was good at always getting sick. But until this program, I realized I'm amazing! Everything I've gone through my whole life, it's incredible! I am a superwoman! I never knew that until this program, until I pushed myself. My disease will never take over my life. I could never thank Dr. Goldner enough, other than doing this video and telling everybody that this does work, because it's real.

Chapter 44
Case Study #19: Barbara's* Story

> *Sjogren's & Lyme In Six Weeks*

Barbara was diagnosed with Sjogren's and Lyme disease. The Sjogren's was causing so much pain in her eyes that she could not deal with any light hitting her eyes, she literally had to put foil over her windows and even with the foil on the windows she had to wear sunglasses indoors, because light hurt her eyes so much. She couldn't go out in the daylight anymore, which meant she couldn't keep up with her friendships and she could no longer go to work, and she loved her job. She is a really powerful woman who had a powerful job and she stopped being able to work, which was a big blow to her. Barbara first tried using Skype consultations with me and even though I gave her very detailed instructions she just couldn't get it right, so she decided to jump into the group to see if I could help her get it right, and you know that I did.

She's a sweet soul and she's also a singer and one of her favorite things to do is to sing for her church. She started getting progressive inflammation and pain in her airway, and stopped being able to sing and could barely talk. She told me was if she could have one thing back, even if she couldn't see in the sunlight again, even if she couldn't work again, she wanted to be able to sing.

Barbara is such an inspiring person; in spite of all the things she's lost, how much pain she was in, and how exhausted she was, she was a positive spirit who encouraged everyone in the group even while she was struggling with getting herself healthy.

She was also very underweight when she started the program. A lot of people think that eating raw foods will make you lose weight, so they hesitate to do the program if they are under-weight, or try to add foods that they think will keep their weight up even if it is off plan. This logic doesn't hold up. While people who eat this way tend to lose weight if they are overweight, people who are underweight will usually end up gaining weight, and people who are light but at a healthy weight will remain within a few pounds of their starting weight. The other reason this isn't really a problem is that weight is NOT an indicator of health from inflammatory illness. If you eat until you are full all day, your body will find a healthy weight.

Your healthy weight is your weight when you are healthy.

If you're underweight from chronic illness and you go on this program you aren't going to just lose weight because you're getting raw vegetables. I've had multiple people that were under 100 pounds when they started the program, who ended up over a hundred pounds by the end of the program. They got healthier and stronger; they could move more, eat more, and continue to gain weight and be healthy. Barbara was 97 pounds when she started the group, and was 104 pounds six weeks later. She would exercise using her body weight in her home.

When the group ended, she was able to have the lights on in her home without needing any sunglasses. She was feeling stronger, no longer in pain. And even more excited, she could sing again. She actually surprised me by sending me a video describing her experience in the group, and at the end she sang Amazing Grace. It was her first time singing since her symptoms had gotten worse, and she sounded like an angel. I watched it with my husband, and we were sobbing watching it. To this day, I can't watch it without crying happy tears. Truly, the best part of my job is witnessing people come back to life, literally into the light from the darkness, and find happiness again the way Barbara did.

Here is what Barbara had to say at the end of the six weeks:

> Hi everybody my name is Barbara and I'm super excited to be here and share my testimony about the last six weeks of my life that have to do with Dr. Goldner's hyper-nourishing healing program. I am a changed person and I hope that I can share with those of you who are possibly considering doing this, those of you who are struggling and suffering with disease, with autoimmune disease, or whatever disease. I have Sjogren's and Lyme, I was diagnosed with those two, and I was terrified. I was looking for something else other than conventional doctors and pills and side effects and all that craziness. I was just hoping that there would be something out there that would be able to help me.

I got on the internet and I searched seriously and I found a testimony of a gentleman who said his Sjogren's was reversed by Dr. G. and I didn't know whether to believe it was true or not but I went for it, and I'll tell you six weeks later my life has changed.

I'm going to dedicate a song, I haven't sang in a long time. My lungs were affected and this is the first time that I've really been able to sing, so I'm going to dedicate this to Dr. G. and everybody that I work with. I consider them my second family, called Amazing Grace. (sings)

Amazing Grace. How sweet the sound That saved a wretch like me I once was lost, but now am found. Was blind but now I see. And you know I was blind, I was blind I was sitting in a dark house for three months without light. When I turned a light on just barely, I had to put on sunglasses because of the photosensitivity from these diseases, and now I have the lights on bright...and my glasses off and I feel so good, I feel so good.

And I hope that whoever is watching this and is hesitant about this, who doesn't quite think it might be right, I remember those feelings of thinking maybe this is just all a fake or fraud. It's not. I'm living proof that when you put the right things in your body, when you put healing foods into your body, it will change and it will heal.

And so, I'm hoping, I'm hoping that my life here that I share with you, just these past six weeks that I've shared of my life will touch someone out there and you'll decide to do this.

There is so much hope and I'm so excited that I feel good and I just want the best for everybody, and I want everybody to be able to experience what I experienced. So, I thank you for letting me share and God bless everybody.

* Name was changed to protect identity.

Chapter 45
Case Study #20: Ashley Lawther's Story

Goodbye Psoriatic Arthritis

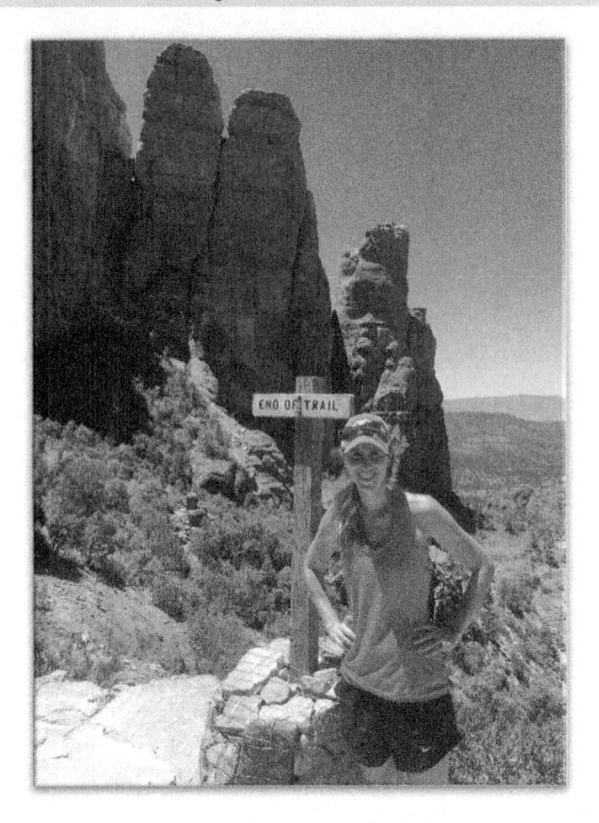

THIS IS AN AFTER PHOTO TAKEN IN JUNE 2019. I COULD HIKE ALL DAY THIS TIME WITH NO PAIN! OPPOSITE OF THE PRIOR YEAR. PHOTO TAKEN IN SEDONA.

Ashley was diagnosed with psoriatic arthritis in 2009. She had back pain, hand and shoulder pain, and foot pain. It made it difficult to do the daily tasks she needed to do as a mom. She also had severe gut pain that hurt so badly she would fall over or faint from the pain.

> I am so excited to share my story, I just finished Dr. Goldner's program. My name is Ashley and I have psoriatic arthritis. I've had joint pain since I was 8 years old and then I was eventually diagnosed when I was 32.
>
> My disease started getting progressively worse, I was having to double up on my medication and even that was not cutting the pain. I couldn't run, I was having difficulty walking, and I was having trouble cooking and doing the dishes. So, I am a mom and I've got 2 kids 11 and 13 and I was just having a hard time doing the "mom things" that I normally would do, and so my husband was having to do that.
>
> These stomach pain attacks would last for about an hour, they were very debilitating where I would sometimes almost pass out from the pain. I'd already gone to two doctors, I had an MRI done, it was inconclusive and then I was going to have to go to another doctor.
>
> I'm only 40 years old and I don't like these limitations that were happening in my life. I want to just be able to go out like most people and just go do things. So, I knew I needed to do something different and so I signed up with Dr. Goldner.
>
> Within 30 days my joint pain was significantly better. And then by the end of the program I could say I have no more joint pain. You know I can run no problem, I have no problem walking. Actually, we took our daughter to an amusement park with some of her friends one night and I walked around for a few hours... normally my body would be kind of hurting afterwards, and then I probably want to wear tennis shoes. Well, this time I didn't wear tennis shoes I just wore flip flops, (and) I felt fine the whole time and that was amazing.
>
> My stomach pain also completely went away. I lost about 10 pounds. My nails are very long and I feel really good. It feels so nice not to just like wake up in the morning and you're body feels so good. Like you can move, you can move freely, nothing hurts. And I can't even remember when the last time I was probably completely pain free, because I dealt with pain since I was little. But I would say probably before I had kids and that was like 13 years ago.

> So, I'm very excited. I was very surprised at how much I grew mentally, and I feel I wasn't expecting that from the program. And I feel like I could weather any type of storm like I'm so strong mentally now. I'm going to keep staying on the program and I definitely recommend that you all check it out and try it out.... I'm very grateful that I did. I'm so glad I was part of the group. I would not have been able to do this on my own even though I would know how to do it. I will guarantee I would have cheated on my own! I asked her a bunch of questions and it was so helpful like I wouldn't have been able to do that if I had done this on my own. I'm so happy I did this and I would definitely recommend this for you all as well.

Like so many of my other clients, Ashley wasn't even hoping for the ability to run and feel amazing, she was just hoping to be able to do the basic things she needed to do, like washing dishes or walking around. Thanks to her dedication to the protocol, she got so much more than that. She is literally glowing with health, and has no limitations anymore.

Chapter 46
Case Study #21: Ellen Jaffe Jones Story

Goodbye Psoriatic Arthritis

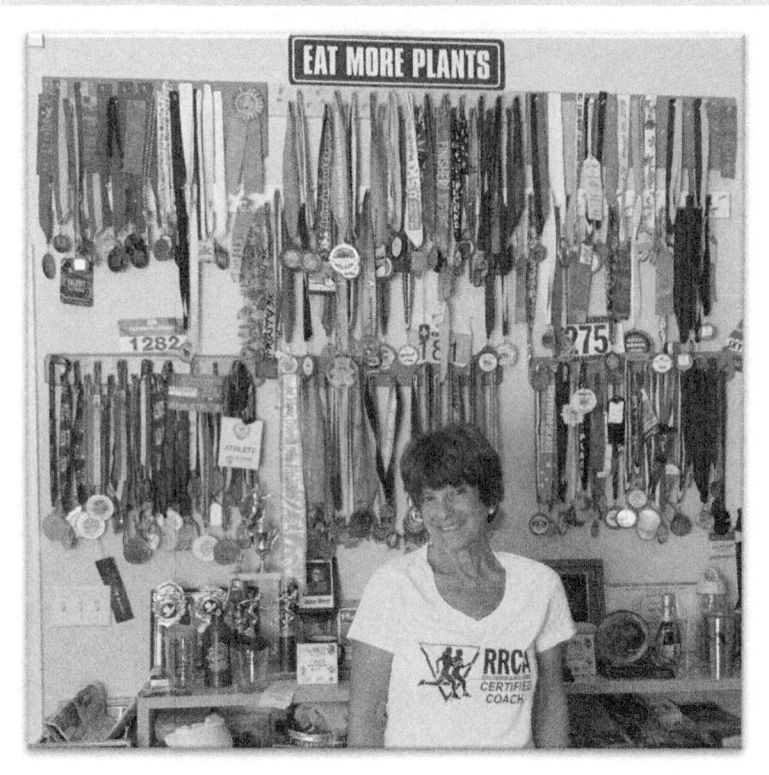

Ellen, whose name you might recognize from the foreword of this book, had a rapid recovery from psoriatic arthritis which developed in spite of years of being on a plant-based diet and being very athletic.

Ellen first changed her diet in her late 20s after a life-threatening colon blockage landed her in the hospital. She started with a macrobiotic diet, then vegetarian, and ultimately vegan. She also started running. While she did well at running and watched her diet carefully, she still struggled with weight. She tried the Atkin's plan for weight loss in the late 90s, which uses high meat and saturated fats and low carbohydrates much like the modern day ketogenic diet. She lost weight, but developed hemorrhaging fibroids. She switched back to vegan, which stopped the fibroids. She says she was "solidly vegan" since 2003.

In the early 2000s she started teaching food demonstrations for plant-based doctors to help the masses learn how to eat healthy foods. She taught them what she learned: to eat a whole-food plant-based diet that is rich in whole grains, vegetables, fruits, and minimized any fats at all.

This is very common in the plant-based community at large, to deter people from eating all fats, even healthy fats like avocados are essential fats like omega-3 fatty acids. I have even heard a well known plant-based doctor incorrectly but forcefully declare that omega-3s can contribute to body fat. This is a dangerous thing to say: first of all omega-3 fatty acids do not become body fat. What they do become is an essential component in your cellular membranes and are vital to the correct functioning of cells. They are also an essential component of neurons in your brain and nervous system, and they are the key ingredients to create your anti-inflammatory immune system. Without ingesting omega-3 fatty acids, you become deficient, because your body cannot synthesize them on its own like other fats. Most people are extremely deficient in omega-3s, which causes an inability to reverse inflammation, heal from disease, lose weight or gain muscle, and also has a negative effect on brain functions like mood and memory.

There is also no emphasis on the importance of raw vegetables, or the importance of eating more vegetables than fruit for disease recovery in a general plant-based diet. Thus, there is a large discrepancy in the results people achieve when they start eating plant-based, depending on which foods they prefer to eat; for example, salads versus rice in beans. The former will accelerate healing, the latter does not.

There is also no attention paid to hydration levels, which has been essential for my clients achieving rapid disease-reversal.

Still, for most people, any whole-food plant-based diet is better than the diet they were previously on, and since there are no inflammatory foods like meat, dairy, processed foods, or oils, there is no inflammation introduced though the diet and people usually feel a lot better and get remission of many symptoms.

What I have found over the years through my clients, is that some people who already have autoimmune disease do not get complete remission or reversal of their disease on a typical whole-food plant-based diet as I just described, and others who have been plant-based for many year develop autoimmune disease even though they were already on a plant-based diet.

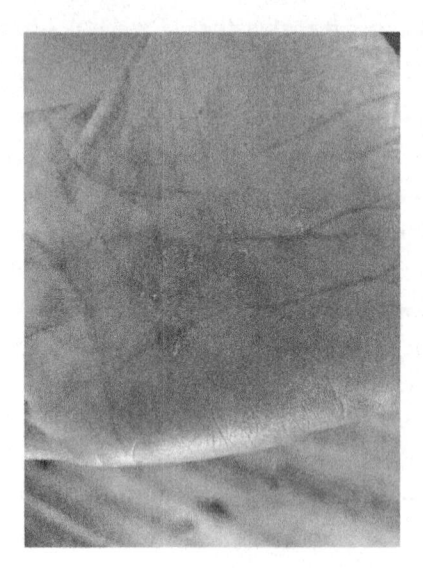

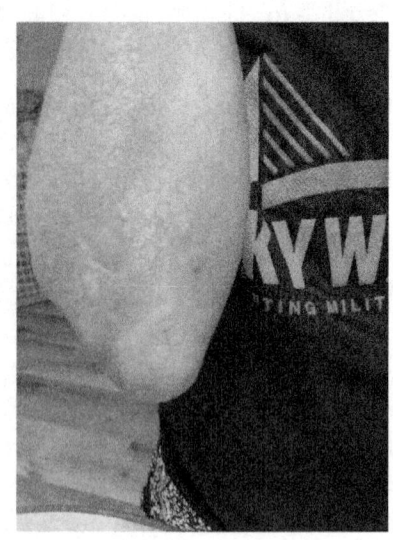

BEFORE HAND BEFORE ELBOW

This causes a great amount of distress, since plant-eaters are under the impression that they won't get sick. I reassure them, as I did Ellen, that if they had been eating meat or dairy they most likely would have gotten sick many years earlier. Not eating inflammatory foods slows it down, but ultimately it is not enough for some people to reverse or avoid autoimmune disease. Their diet wasn't making them sick, but it wasn't anti-inflammatory enough. The answer is hyper-nourishment.

When I met with Ellen, she did admit that she had added some processed food in the form of vegan protein bars recently, especially on the road, which definitely contributed inflammation. She was also not getting any omega-3s, almost no raw vegetables, and was only drinking 64 ounces of water a day.

In the winter of 2018, Ellen noticed that her hands were getting red and white flaky plaques on them and her nails were starting to come off. Her fingers were swollen and stiff. Her energy was fading and she was leaning on caffeine to get through her day.

She went to the doctor and he diagnosed her with psoriatic arthritis, the same illness that crippled her father. Ellen was devastated. She set up an appointment with a rheumatologist and then asked her friend, Dr. Joel Kahn, a vegan cardiologist, what he thought. He immediately referred her to me. I got her started on hyper-nourishment, with all healing foods from smoothies and salads until remission of her symptoms, and then she added back some cooked plant-based unprocessed foods in addition to keeping up her daily smoothies and water over 100 ounces a day.

Within 2 weeks of hyper-nourishment, her hands were back to normal – no more swelling or pain, and rashes were gone too. By the time she got to the rheumatologist (6 months later), the doctor was confused as to why she was there because she had "no signs of inflammation". Not only did the inflammation, pain, and rashes go away, but Ellen lost 15lbs without any extra effort because the nourishment increased her metabolism. Her athletic performance has also gone up: she is beating her old best running times by 5 minutes even though she is older now.

Ellen is incredibly grateful and open about her healing journey. She has posted about it online and she even included a slide about me in each of her recent talks. When I met her at a recent conference, she kept introducing me as "the doctor that saved my life." Ellen is a joy to be around, her enthusiasm for life and for health is infectious. Here is what she wanted to share with you:

> I thought my life was over when I was diagnosed with the autoimmune disease, psoriatic arthritis. From what I read online, I would be lucky to be running in a year, let alone walking. I would be in excruciating pain and forget about even getting out of bed until taking medicine which should be kept at bedside. How could this have possibly happened to a healthy vegan?
>
> My dad was an awesome tennis player. He used to play with me through childhood into high school. Somewhere in his 60's, arthritis set in and by the end of his life at 93, he had arthritis so bad he could barely walk. His toes and fingers were swollen and curled. I remembered that he used a tar shampoo for psoriasis on his scalp,

which I would later learn often accompanies psoriatic arthritis. He suffered painfully from heart disease and diabetes. I figured, "I'm vegan. None of that will happen to me." I vaguely took notice that along with me, my dad, oldest sister her daughter had psoriasis on their elbows, too. That same sister was diagnosed with arthritis in her twenties, most likely psoriatic arthritis, although many forms of arthritis were lumped together back then. Another lovely family gene, we joked.

I sometimes joke (to deal with the pain) that my family may have been the sickest family in America. In total, there were 4 breast cancers in my family: My mom, aunt and both sisters. My oldest sister, eleven years older than me, got diabetes in her twenties, which developed into heart disease and heart by-passes in her forties. My other sister, nine years older than me, got breast cancer for the first time in her thirties and would endure a poor quality of life getting it two more times. My aunt got it in the 1950's in her thirties and died six months later in our home where she and her daughter who was a year older than me, had come to live. I was five at the time. The night my aunt died, my cousin and I clung to each other to sleep. We tried to drown out the crying and wailing we heard in the other rooms. The trauma never left us.

My oldest sister became obese and underwent surgery in her 60's for a "routine" herniated disc. With her diabetic compromised immune system, MRSA or methicillin-resistant Staphylococcus aureus, a bacterium with antibiotic resistance, entered her blood somehow through the sterile IV, lodged in her neck and made her a paraplegic in a nursing home for the rest of her 6 miserable years of life. At least breast cancer waited to strike until her final year on the planet. She had a double mastectomy, one prophylactically, which she had been considering for much of her life.

As a 2-time Emmy-winning TV investigative reporter, figuring out the truth about food became the investigative reporting job of my life. At age 28, I almost died of a colon blockage. I collapsed in the TV station's bathroom and 2 friends had to help me into the car to drive me to the emergency room. Doctors said they had never seen a colon blockage so large in someone so young and that I would need to be on medicine and stool softeners the rest of my life. That pain was the worst...worse than natural childbirth three times. I ran to the health food store and read all 5 books on fiber. That's all there was at the time. At first, like many of at the time, I chose a macrobiotic diet which was widely touted to prevent cancer. The progression after that was vegetarian, then vegan. I was quoted in a newspaper article about my TV career, "I'm not a health nut," I defended under a photo of me standing in front of all my whole grains and beans described as "food stuffs." But I totally was. My sisters proclaimed I was crazy, a member of a cult and I was never invited to family functions again unless my dad insisted upon it.

My parents got it. My dad, who used to have a constant sinus infection and even avoided serving in World War II because he couldn't breathe out of a gas mask, got his assisted living facility to serve soy milk. He was astounded that his life-long habit of expectorating (coughing and spitting) on sidewalks went away almost overnight.

For many, giving up dairy is like turning off a constantly running faucet in the throat. Because my collapse at the TV station was so public, I began educating my co-workers about fiber. I'll never forget that the on-air pharmacist, who was a pharmacist in real life, couldn't get over how much increasing fruit and vegetables changed his life-long constipation. The word "vegan" hadn't made it into the newsroom yet.

I started running in my twenties. I had battled weight since childhood not knowing that my family's love of Italian restaurants, ice cream and living a block from the best bakery in St. Louis was probably the culprit. A morning without gooey butter cake was like a morning without sunshine. On a recent visit to my hometown, I was astounded to see that although the bakery was long closed, coffee shops still carry the cake and derivatives such as gooey butter cookies. A recent newspaper story mocked St. Louis "traditional" foods but was clear about how unhealthy they were. Do we not get this yet?

I was trying to avoid the family breast cancer scourge. My OBGYN told me that a low-fat diet would help keep my weight down which was critical in avoiding breast cancer. He, and other doctors said, "You better do things differently or you'll end up like everyone else in your family." I took their advice to heart. In high school, I tried the first high-protein Stillman diets, which were the precursor to Atkins, which I would also do. It worked, as high protein diets often do, but at the expense of the heart and kidneys.

As I yo-yo dieted, losing and gaining back the same 30 pounds, my cholesterol topped at 203 and doctors were ready to put me on Lipitor.

On a 5'3" frame, those 30 pounds slowed me down and had an impact. It's important to understand that in the early days, doctors didn't have access to the information and research we do now. Consumers didn't have access to the science like we do now on social media. I had a few zig zags such as the time I was pregnant and both doctors and nurses said I needed to include whey protein in my diet to improve brain function of my unborn children. That was a heavy. Who wouldn't listen to a doctor if he or she was promising brain damage if you didn't feed your developing fetus the right foods. Fortunately, we now know that a balanced, healthful vegan diet is appropriate for all stages of life, including pregnancy. I would eventually find my way back to veganism with no diversions.

Running was an easy way to keep the weight under control. I didn't begin racing seriously until my 50's, when I was solidly vegan. I often joked that I'd win my age group because at my age, I could just show up. Lately, that hasn't been as true as the Boomers retire and hire full-time professional coaches. As of this writing, I have placed in 173 5K or longer races since 2006 "just" on plants. I don't place in every race I do. So I've probably raced in at least another 50 without placing but still wearing the vegan message shirt.

I received a gold medal at the 2019 National Senior Games in the W65-69 4x100 meters and placed 10th in the US in the 1500 and 800 meters. I've competed at Nationals in 2017 and 2013 and also placed in the top 10 in similar events. I've done 2 marathons and 13 half marathons. I never really intended to compete so much, but other runners who suddenly had nutrition degrees, would stand next to me while I had my award medal in my hand wearing my bright Eat Vegan on $4 a Day running singlet and say, "You can't run/race on a vegan diet." So it became an act of defiance and an effort to prove them wrong. At my first Nationals in 2013, a woman who placed first in our age group came up to me before the 1500 meters and said, "Ellen Jaffe Jones, cookbook author, right?" I said, "Yes...who are you, and how and why do you know that?" She quipped, "I study all my competition." I thought, "Whoa, I'm so out of my league. I'm just a weekend athlete who doesn't train much." I would learn that many of these women hire coaches from UCLA and other universities, and even paid for their coaches to attend the games with them. I attributed doing as well as I did to a vegan diet.

In another act of defiance, one of my hot buttons is the wretched post-race food. I have seen such absurd sights as Sarasota Memorial Hospital allowing Duncan Donuts to be the title sponsor of a 5K race. My dream in life, after 40 years of running and racing, to cross a finish line and not have to inhale charred animal remains. At many races, the only vegan post-race food was a banana. The reason races have food is that ideally, you should consume protein and carbohydrates within the first hour after intense exercise to rebuild muscle tissues and micro-tears that are a normal part of exertion. At one such race, when I hopped up on the first place podium, I held up my defiant arm with a banana in hand. Not long after, as a board member of our local running club, I arranged to be the title sponsor with the only condition that it have all vegan post-race food. They happily agreed, and I spent another wad of money and went and bought enough vegan food from a health food store to feed the army that shows up at these races. I was told by PCRM and No Meat Athlete that this was the first time in the US that a large, long-standing, mainstream 5K went vegan. The 15th annual Boo Run was totally vegan and handed out carrots at the finish line (which I also delivered) to every finisher, replacing the insidious chocolate milk cartons paid for by the Dairy Council's well-publicized campaign, "Marketing Chocolate Milk to Children as the Ideal Recovery Drink." I can't tell you how many times this happens at races when it's challenging to find enough water. The meat industry pays for teams to compete and wear their shirts at races. They were out in force at the National Senior Games wearing "Beef Loving Texans," and "Fueled by Beef." There is not doubt this is in response to vegan athletes outperforming in their vegan shirts. My hope was that this vegan race would be copied elsewhere.

These were challenging times to figure out nutrition wisdom. But to lower my cholesterol, I went vegan and it dropped to 140 by the next blood test. All was good until I began working as a financial consultant for Smith Barney where we had no choice except the pizza topping at working lunches and salads at Morton's Steakhouse, where many company client dinners were held. I kept McDougall soup cups under my desk. At a sedentary job, my lipids and weight shot up again. My once 120 pound scale reading was 150. The Atkins diet was enjoying a newfound media blitz. The New York Times, in the 2002 controversial Gary Taubs article, "What If It's All Been A Big Fat Lie" made me think the science had changed. Atkins was on all the talk and news shows. I was desperate to lose the weight. But this time, the weight didn't seem to budge. What I would later learn is that the science hadn't changed, only the marketing had. Atkins had heart disease when he died, and the Stillman, Zone, South Beach and Keto diets all had the same high-protein ring. I'd read and tried them all.

Finally, I quit Smith Barney and began media consulting. I contacted Physicians Committee for Responsible Medicine and asked if they needed media training. President Dr. Neal Barnard, who I had heard speak in the 90's, was eloquent by birth, but he most graciously said he was considering media training for his staff and anyone else interested in being a spokesperson. That began a wonderful relationship of flying to Washington and training. On one visit, I smelled my way into the kitchen and was told that the first recipes for the first program to teach the masses how to cook and eat vegan were being developed. It was called The Cancer Project and is now part of PCRM's Food for Life program. Since I'd been informally trying to teach anyone I met how to eat this way, I signed up for the training and taught free cooking classes, sometimes as many as 2 a day 5 days a week, for 6 years.

In 2008, I began thinking if we could show the world how cheap it is to eat vegan on a budget, we would have many more vegans. Having been a TV consumer and investigative reporter, I was familiar with the Consumer Price Index and knew how inexpensive whole foods were. I got tired of the news stories that said you couldn't eat well on food stamps, and I crunched the numbers on my favorite recipes and wrote Eat Vegan on $4 a Day. It took years to get it published, but by 2011, the book was in print and for the first time starting that year, Google searches for "vegan" started overtaking "vegetarian," The world was starting to listen.

So the question begs asking, how does such a healthy vegan athlete get an autoimmune disease? Aren't vegans supposed to be poster children and bulletproof? Indeed, I have been called a vegan poster child for health. I believe I still am. It's pretty simple how it happened.

As typically driven people do, I wasn't content to just appear for a book talk and vanish. My first Vegfest speaking gig was the 2011 Toronto Vegfest. At the time, it was the largest Vegfest in North America. At Smith Barney, I learned to spend all day at a table trying to acquire clients. I applied the same principles to Vegfests. I figured that if my publisher was paying my hotel, airfare, the best vegan meals on the planet and royalties, the least I could do was stay at the table through each day of the Vegfest and help sell not only my books, but all the other books as well, especially since I'd read most of them. Much to my shock, he had never had an author do that before. We bonded and I would end up writing 5 more books during the next 6 years.

In addition to staying at the table all day, I would help my publisher unload, set up, and do inventory and pack up at the end of Vegfests, it made for long days. I loved it. As a result, I would skip lunch in favor of my stash of Lara Bars or later, Cliff Bars. As I like to say now, I'm a recovering Cliff Bar addict. It was a stressful lifestyle, especially coupled with the challenges of flying. One time, my flight to the Nashville Vegfest was cancelled on my way to the airport. I had no choice but to reroute the car and start driving the 800 miles and 14 hours to Nashville to make it time for my talk the next day.

In the winter of 2018, I started feeling pain in some of my fingers and noticing that my joints were not only stiff and swollen upon waking, but there were crusty outbreaks at the joints, not unlike the psoriasis and white "plaques" that had been on my elbow much of my adult life. But it got stranger. My fingernails were starting to come off! It was classic psoriatic arthritis. The white nail tips were no longer just tips. Their borders became increasingly large and irregular. My normally high-octane energy was fading. I was tired. Lethargic. I thought, how can I possibly keep up my travel schedule, running and continuing what I'm doing? I read more online. I could only find one other person who had been diagnosed with psoriatic arthritis who wrote on the psoriatic arthritis website about his tough journey trying to continue running. Most other Google searches assured me I probably wouldn't die of the disease, but running would most likely be a past memory. My life would become excruciatingly painful every waking minute. My primary doctor and an allergist said it looked like psoriatic arthritis. I visited alternative and functional medicine doctors. One wanted me to spend thousands of dollars for chelation therapy. It was risky as the studies validating this were scarce. I went to a stem cell replacement doctor who said I really wasn't a candidate for that.

I made an appointment with a rheumatologist. The soonest I could get in was 6 months out. In the meantime, I was boo-hooing to my co-author on Vegan Sex, cardiologist and the amazing, generous-with-his-time, Dr. Joel Kahn. He said, "You should talk to Dr. Brooke

Goldner. She's really busy with so many people needing and getting her wonderful help, but let's see what we can do." Dr. Goldner would later tell me that he left her a brief message that said only, "Fix her."

I bought Dr. Goldner's books and scheduled an online consult with her. It was the best money I have ever paid for anything. What became painfully clear is that I was subsisting on Cliff Bars and in the process forgot about those daily greens. Autoimmune diseases usually strike in the twenties and thirties. I was lucky to have mine hit in my 60's, which both Dr. Goldner and I believe was a result of my healthy diet and lifestyle up until I hit the road on book tour. Runners, vegan or not, are generally known to have better immune systems than the population at large. Although I know plenty of runners who extol the virtues of butter and bacon believing that running is an insurance policy against disease. It is not. I've known runners to get heart disease, cancer and in some cases, diabetes.

Dr. Goldner suggested the ultimate fast track, the Rapid Recovery Plan. It was all raw: smoothies, salads, fancy raw vegan dishes plus optional tofu. Sleep was mandatory. Guilty on all counts of being weak in that area too. My social media became so popular with my books that my publisher asked me to be their social media director for a while to try to clone what I had done for myself for their other authors. Eventually, with 6 books out, I had to bail on that and soon hired a virtual assistant I still pay to help with my own social media, among other things.

The key to recovery and keeping the immune system in check was the green smoothies and 100 ounces, that's a gallon of water a day. According to Dr. Goldner, at least that amount is needed to reverse inflammation and energize.

Dr. Goldner is very methodical and precise about her smoothies. Bless her, she even asks her followers to send/post pictures of their smoothies to make sure they've got it right.

Here's the magic formula: Grind ½ cup of flax seeds, or a flax/chia mix fresh daily in a high-powered blender, like a Vitamix. Then stuff that blender all the way to the top with kale, spinach, collard greens and whatever fruit, such as a pear, a banana or two and whatever liquid you want...almond milk, water etc. to blend and make the medicine go down. Additional greens could come in the form the cruciferous veggies like broccoli, cabbage and cauliflower in smoothies, salads or snacks.

To this day, even well after my symptoms resolved, I prepare a huge, blender-full smoothie that fills 3 glasses daily or every other day.

Here's the deal. I really thought my life, especially my running life was done. I had spent my life dedicated to the cause of health, and of course, so intimately intertwined with the environment and animals. The diagnosis made me feel like a failure and that I had let many down. Entire generations were losing each other on the standard American diet and didn't even know it. I didn't want to be part of that equation. My parents were so sick and diseased by the time I had children, they couldn't lift them, let alone babysit. How I had wanted it to be different for my daughters.

I don't know who said this first, but it applies here: Genes load the gun, food pulls the trigger. I was so depressed by what I read online, especially initially, I cried. Dr. Goldner advised, "Stop Googling, Ellen! Those horror stories you're reading online are from non-vegans who didn't come into this with all the advantages you did. Their outcome may not be at all what yours can be." Dr. Goldner was SO reassuring and kind in all of her conversations with me, whether they were in emails, texts or on the phone.

The most bizarre part of the recovery is how quickly the fingernails started improving. You think of fingernails as taking weeks and months to grow just a tiny bit. But the jagged edges of where the white nails met the pink fingernail bed began improving almost immediately. I know the recovery was well below the skin. But skin is the largest organ we own, and it is a clear mirror into the soul of our immune system health. I shared the before and after photos on social media. They were dramatic, I thought, until I saw some of Dr. Goldner's photos she posted of other incredible results.

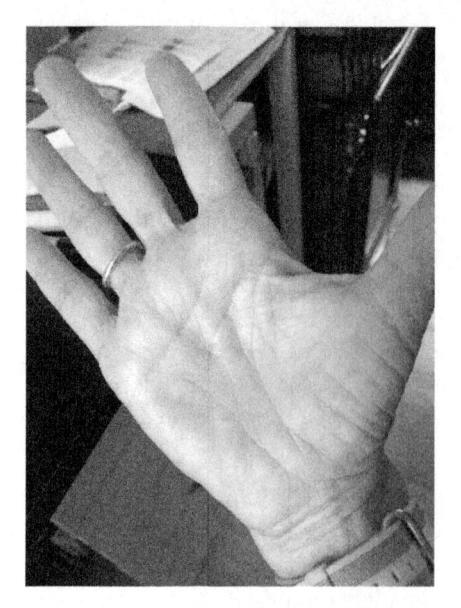

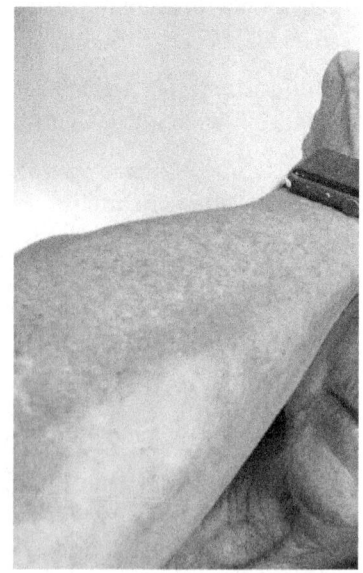

AFTER HAND   AFTER ELBOW

I know many vegans who are in it solely or mostly for the animals. So am I. I began protesting circuses when my babes, now in their thirties, were literally still in arms. I get it. If vegan food was the most unhealthiest food in the world, many of us would eat it anyway to save an animal or the planet. But the good news is, there are many foods that are the healthiest the planet has to offer. If I have to choose between a vegan hotdog or donut and a kale smoothie, the smoothie wins every time. While some vegans say nothing matters as long as food is vegan, the goal, it seems to me, ought to be that we enjoy good health to add extra years to promote the vegan message. It is important that as activists, we have all the strength and energy we can. We're no good for the animals and the planet if we can't bound out of bed every morning with purpose, drive and determination. The planet and the animals have no time for us to discuss it some more and get it right. The time is now.

It was almost a year to the day from my diagnosis when I competed and won the gold at the National Senior Games. Since my recovery, I had placed in many more 5K races, races I thought I would never do. I kept that appointment with the rheumatologist who couldn't believe I ever had psoriatic arthritis, even though I had provided before and after photos as part of my medical record. She squeezed or touched joints on my extremities. She said, "You don't have any signs of inflammation anywhere on your body. Why are you here?" "I guess you don't get too many patients like me." I gave her my best smile. "I'm sorry, not sorry I cured myself before the 6 month wait to see you was up. I thought you might like to see that." She was very businesslike, curt and made little eye contact, instead typing constantly on her laptop like an overworked, stressed doctor. I showed her Dr. Goldner's book, but she showed no interest in it other than a cursory, "Hmmmm…." But that was OK. I had scanned and printed the book cover and included it in my medical records just in case she got curious later.

Right after that clean bill of health appointment, I ran one of the most challenging races: a 10K (6.2 miles) over Tampa Bay's Sunshine Skyway Bridge. It's 2 miles up and 2 miles down at a 4% grade with a mile on either side of that. It is one of the longest and highest US bridges. If I had not stopped to take a picture with my phone at the top, I would have placed third in my age group instead of eighth. I missed it by a second. But I was glad to have preserved the exhilarating memory from the pinnacle of that somewhat scary bridge.

A week after running my heart out at the National Senior Games, my dream came true of running a 5K with my daughters for the first time. They arranged it and included their significant others. To add more sweetness, we all placed in our age groups in a competitive large city race.

One of the most amazing things that happened while doing the protocol was that in the first 3 months, I lost 15 pounds. I wasn't even trying. I started at 138 and today it is 123. Much to my surprise, my 5K times have improved by 5 minutes over a year ago. I did nothing different in my training. If anything, I cut back more to rest. My 10K and half marathon times improved significantly as well. That's not supposed to happen as we age. It's known that weight loss can have this kind of effect on racing times, making you faster. I feel strong, energized and all while giving up even occasional alcohol and my beloved coffee, since both can be psoriatic arthritis triggers.

As I'm fond of saying #runningismyactivism. At every race where I wear a vegan message shirt, other runners, their families and friends see the message. I encourage you to sign up for these, even if you only walk as many do, just to wear those message shirts. If you should place in your age group, the professional race photographers will be taking your picture and it will end up on many websites. Everybody else who places in your age group will be taking pictures or having their friends and families take pictures that will end up all over social media too. They might happen to see that a runner wearing a vegan message on their shirt placed too. Maybe even first place. Maybe they also had the misconception that vegans are weak or can't race. It is a great way to plunge our message into the mainstream and to reach deniers.

Dr. Goldner gave me my life back. There is no finer gift than health, and for that, I will always be forever grateful.

Chapter 47
Case Study #22: Rose La Fond's Story

Hypothyroid, Binge Eating, & Polycystic Ovarian Syndrome In Six Weeks

Rose joined my 6 week rapid recovery group desperate for relief from hypothyroid, Polycystic Ovarian Syndrome (PCOS), binge eating, pain and weakness. Rose prefers to be referred to by neutral pronouns like they, their and them rather then he or she so I will discuss Rose's story using those pronouns.

Rose had constant pain from their back and legs. They also had painful rashes on their arms that hurt so badly they couldn't wear long sleeves. They were weak and tired. They also had severe abdominal pains. At only 26 years old, they were disabled and unable to work or go to school. Even though they had supportive parents and a loyal partner, they felt like their life was about pain and loss. The constant abdominal pain caused Rose to feel suicidal; they couldn't imagine continuing to live a life in constant pain. These thoughts were terrifying.

They worked hard and followed our daily advice and support in the group. They communicated their fears and symptoms and appreciated the daily support and assignments we gave them to work on their emotional health along with their physical health.

After only six weeks, Rose truly felt like a new person. They had energy, was building up strength, felt less anxious and happier, and most importantly, hopeful that they had a life worth living.

Rose has already lowered their thyroid medicine three times since the group because their thyroid function keeps going up. They are now on half the dose they were on when they started the group a couple months ago. Rose no longer has painful periods, and is exercising and enjoying life more. They also felt no urges to binge while in the group, which was a big victory for them.

Rose has a huge heart and was such a joy to have in the group. They were always encouraging fellow group members even as they worked towards their own healing. I am so proud of you Rose!

Rose was so excited about how much better they felt after six weeks, and immediately made a video about their recovery to share. This is what they said.

> My name is Rose La Fond, I started trying to do the protocol by myself August 31st of 2018, and I obviously was not doing it, quite right… I started the program, the six-week program October 6th. So, I was diagnosed with hypothyroidism, I don't remember how long ago. Hashimoto's, polycystic ovarian syndrome, PCOS, sporadic urticaria, hives that don't seem to be tied to anything. Multiple types of dermatitis, a binge-eating disorder, and arthritis with sciatica, though they haven't been able to diagnose what kind of arthritis. And then undiagnosable but serious gut episodes, gut pain… The gastroenterologist and allergist figured it's autoimmune, but I've never tested positive for autoimmune disorder, normal CRP, normal Sed rate, no ANAs. And I don't know, they could still be autoimmune, it's what makes the most sense. I have other autoimmune like eczema and psoriasis, and I know Dr. G says that, sometimes it can take years of having symptoms before you have a positive ANA. And then also kind of undiagnosable food sensitivities to virtually everything.
>
> So, symptoms painful period, pain in every joint especially my spine, coccyx, neck, and lumbar. With the gut pain episodes, I've had gut problems since starting solid food at six months. I finally went to the ER for the first time, June 2016 and they couldn't do anything for me. And that was what I was expecting, which is why I hadn't gone previously.
>
> This past spring, late winter it started getting bad; worse and worse to the point where they had to call the fire department. And I had to go to the ER several times… the gut pain, I would have a rash covering my body, and it started turning into hives. Yeah, other symptoms, one of the rashes is all over my arms. And I think it's been there since I was a baby, but it is covered in pustules and it stings and prickles like needles. So, I've always hated wearing long sleeves, and fatigue and weakness pretty badly.
>
> So, these symptoms have caused me to have to go to a lot of doctors. My parents have spent an enormous amount of money. The gut pain

turned into constant pain over the summer, it just was constant and it's very, very scary. It feels like I want to die, when I have an episode and I can't stop myself from crying in pain.

The arthritis is also very scary, it started, I'm almost 27 and it started when I was almost 20. I mean it started when I was 13, but it really started when I was almost 20, with horrible sciatica. And it's just gotten worse from there, and the only thing that the rheumatologist could recommend was self-injected chemotherapy which I read about and decided not to take. The pain has made me really unable to do a lot, I live on the second floor of an apartment with no elevator and I can't carry my backpack up or down the stairs.

I've had pain for so long, I've never been able to get a driver's license. I've barely been able to work and I've been unable to work for two years, now unemployed. I'm completely financially dependent on my partner and my parents. I'm disabled. I just had to drop out of college for the second time this quarter, which sucks. Disability sucks, but what's even worse than disability is not being able to take the pain. And it's been getting worse and I saw no hope of it getting better.

So, I expected the pain to be so bad after a year or two more that, I just wouldn't be able to take it and I would have to kill myself, which I'm sorry is painful for people to hear. But there's only so much pain I can take before I need relief.

So, since going on the protocol or trying it on my own August 31st, I have had zero hives which is great. I've gone to ER zero times, I had no stomach aches, zero. I had one mild stomach ache during the program.

I stopped binging, I just have no urge to binge anymore. I have zero pain with periods, I was not expecting that, zero, it's like I'm not even having my period. It's amazing, there's not even discomfort, there's no breast pain, no cramping nothing, it's fantastic. And I've lowered my thyroid dose and I have zero discomfort from the rash on my arms, and it's starting to slowly go down.

I'm able to exercise and get stronger, the joint pain is just starting to go down. So, now I'm able to exercise, I'm able to cut soft things with a knife now and make smoothies which I was not able to (do).

I'm not expecting such a short life now. I'm not expecting to die after one or two more years. Dr. G has given me this, she has given me my life back. She's given me a healthy relationship with food. She's given me a healthier relationship with myself. And getting to being in the group I got support and guidance and a community. Dr. G and Thomas Tadlock were there all the time every day all through the day, answering questions, supporting, encouraging. I got help with exercises because I was so scared, every time I had tried doing physical therapy exercises in the past I'd hurt myself and flared up the pain. And really importantly, we got therapy homework and the group really important for me. I have changed a lot; my expectation of the future is the biggest thing that has changed. I'm optimistic now about the future; about my future about my life and I get to look forward to having a future, to having a life. I have gained self-respect and self-pride. I've gained liking myself and who I am, and being proud of and liking taking care of myself and prioritizing myself.

Thank You Dr. G, Thank You Thomas Tadlock. Thank you everyone in the group... I get to live and be happy and get better. Thank you, Dr. G, Thank You Thomas Tadlock, thank you for sharing your protocol with all of us.

Chapter 48
Case Study #23: Whitney Lee's Story

Celiac Disease & Type I Diabetes In Four Weeks

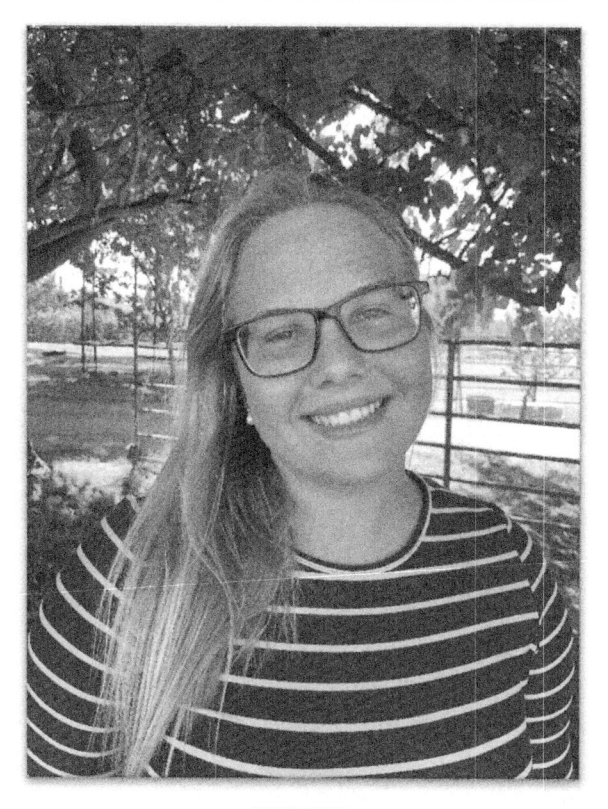

BEFORE

Whitney Lee was a senior in high school when I first met her. She had had type I diabetes (insulin-dependent) since she was a child. She had become accustomed to having diabetes and using insulin to control her blood sugar levels. Her life went into a tailspin when she was diagnosed with celiac disease. She told me, "it's easier to have diabetes than celiac" because she could just take insulin for her blood sugar, but avoiding grains felt so restrictive and almost impossible. She found herself in so much pain from the celiac disease, she would be doubled over in pain, and ended up missing a lot of school, after only eating a little bit of food containing gluten. Her mother took her to the doctor and they confirmed she had celiac disease through blood tests that showed she had the antibodies.

Whitney's mother came to an event I taught with my husband, Amazing Fitness and Health and learned about how my nutrition protocol helped other autoimmune diseases and wondered if it could help her daughter. They decided to try my 4 Week Rapid Recovery program. It was difficult for Whitney, eating a raw diet is hard enough, especially early on when you are having a lot of cravings, it was even more challenging going to high school and being around peers eating cooked food and junk food. She stuck with it and had an amazing turn-around.

She quickly found that in spite of having smoothies that contain fruit, her blood sugars were far lower and she could use a lot less insulin. I have witnessed that happen repeatedly in clients with both type I and type II diabetes, blood sugar goes down. Many people incorrectly believe that carbohydrates and sugars cause diabetes. Current studies indicate that insulin resistance is actually caused by saturated fat from eating meat coating the muscle cells and blocking insulin receptors. That is why there is an increase in blood sugar when the person eats carbohydrates, because insulin cannot bind and tell the cells to absorb the sugars. When a diabetic switches to a plant-based diet, their blood sugars go down dramatically.[25] Whitney also noted that her stomach pain went away and she felt energetic.

Now of course, there won't be symptoms of celiac on a raw vegan diet that has no grains. The question was, would it affect the antibody production and her disease? After the 4 weeks, Whitney got blood tests drawn and she no longer tested positive for celiac. She slowly reintroduced gluten-containing foods and had no negative reaction. She was thrilled. She decided to stay completely plant-based with her green smoothies for nourishment with raw foods and omega-3s, and stayed symptom-free. I ran into her at a conference 2 years after she did Rapid Recovery with me and she was still doing well. She is currently finished up her associate's degree and writes Celiac under "previous medical conditions" because she no longer suffers from the disease. She came to the conference to see me in person and tell me how great she was doing. This is what she had to say for others who are interested in her story:

> I used to have celiac starting my freshman year in high school, and I was just in deep pain, puking a lot, couldn't get out of bed for like a week, every time I had gluten. And so, then I went completely away from wheat and all that but that was kind of really hard in America, because everything has wheat.
>
> Then my mom heard about Dr. Goldner. We got connected and I did the plan. It was very hard for me to do the plan being in high school, but it ended up working very well. It's been I think two years now and I'm still not allergic to gluten, still drinking green smoothies, doing the vegan diet and it's helped a lot. I'm moving along with my life perfectly fine...There's no signs of celiac, blood is free of antibodies, everything's fine. I am celiac free.

I have shared Whitney's story online, with a video of her sharing her experience, and some people got very angry about it, saying "there is no cure for celiac!". It is always interesting to me when someone hears a positive story of disease-recovery and gets angry. I used to encounter that same response when I told people I no longer have lupus. Some people would get excited and hopeful, and others would get angry, as if I was diminishing how sick they were by saying the disease can be reversed with diet and lifestyle. I refrain from using the word cure because it tends to get people into an intellectual conversation about whether or not this is a cure or a remission, rather than focused on the important take-away, which is that no matter what you call it, it's the best thing you can do for yourself! That is why I use the term disease-reversal, because it is completely accurate: the disease started, became chronic, and now has been reversed. That is also why I tell the stories of people's recovery for motivation. You can argue about whether or not you think this is a cure, a remission, or a miracle, but you can't argue with a person's experience. This is Whitney's story, and that is her truth.

For Whitney, she does not test positive for celiac anymore, and does not require treatment or dietary restriction beyond a high raw plant-based diet. I do not recommend that anyone diagnosed with celiac start eating grains without confirming they are well under their doctor's care. I do recommend anyone with celiac to try hyper-nourishment to get the best health possible.

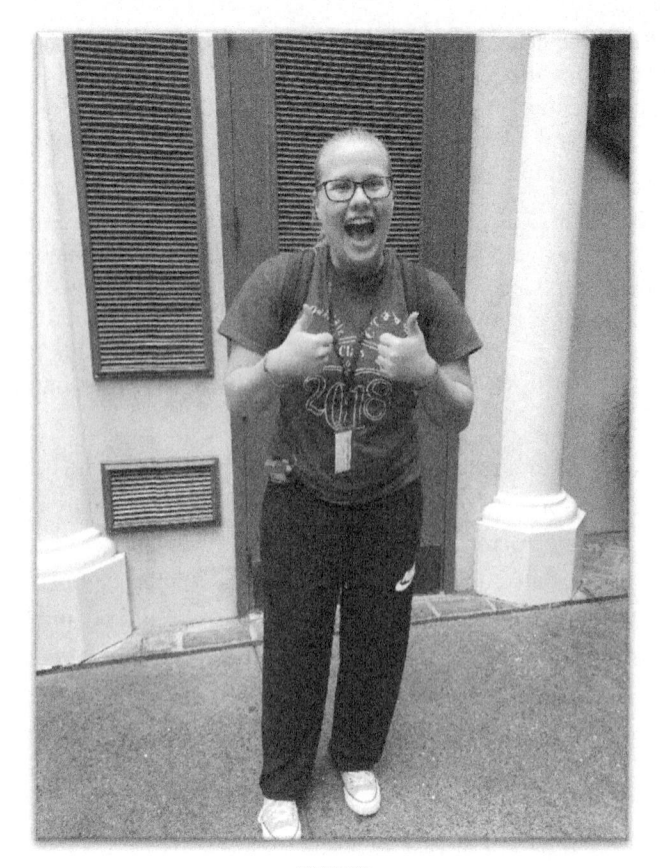

AFTER

Chapter 49
Case Study #24

Non-Alcoholic Fatty Liver Disease & Elevated Liver Enzymes

While I have not had someone come to me specifically to help them with elevated liver enzymes, I have frequently found that people struggling with other illnesses like autoimmune disease, diabetes, and heart disease also have elevated liver enzymes or fatty liver disease.

This may be a function of increased inflammation that is affecting their liver or be caused by their medications. Many people with non-alcoholic fatty liver disease are triggered by high levels of processed sugars in their diets. No matter the cause, I have discovered that the liver rapidly returns to normal functioning with the rapid recovery nutrition plan. The liver has long been known to be efficient at regenerating itself, so it is not surprising that this organ responds so efficiently to an anti-inflammatory nutrition plan. That said, my clients are often shocked to see their liver tests normalize, because their doctors didn't have an explanation or a solution for them, just told them it was a chronic problem they had to live with.

Below are the labs of someone I was treating for lupus and Sjogren's with rapid recovery. She initially was in so much pain, that even at only 21 years old, she had to lay down in her bed just to put her own pants on. She also had chronic pleurisy and had never had a remission since she had been diagnosed. In three weeks, she was able to put her own pants on standing up, had no lung pain, and was playing tennis! Her chronic acne also disappeared. When she got her labs back though, she was most astonished to see her liver had normalized. She had chronic liver inflammation for years before she worked with me. You can see her numbers for her AST liver enzyme elevated at 54 and 56 when tested in 2010 and 2011. After doing 3 weeks of hyper-nourishment with me in 2012, her liver markers dropped to normal and have stayed normal for years afterwards. Her doctors were unsure what was causing the liver inflammation and had no answers for her; maybe it was the medicines, maybe it was the autoimmune disease. They weren't sure. As soon as she got on my Rapid Recovery program, her numbers went back to normal and stayed there.

	05/17/2010	05/19/2011	04/02/2012	10/12/2013	04/09/2014	07/08/2014	03/17/2015	08/28/2015
ALT *(Standard Range 15-65 U/L)*	54	56	29	16	23	19	23	13

I told you about Nir, who was able to reverse his type 2 diabetes in five weeks on rapid recovery also had chronic liver inflammation for 15 years. His doctor didn't know why. Four weeks into the rapid recovery program for his diabetes, his liver function tests were all normal. As you can see from his lab report below, his liver enzymes were high back in 2009, all the way until April 2018 when we started his program.

	09/15/2009	05/10/2011	03/03/2016	12/27/2016	08/01/2017	04/04/2018	05/18/2018
ALT *(Standard Range 15-65 U/L)*	81	87	89	93	98	78	**50**
AST *(Standard Range 0-36 U/L)*	41	46	45	49	40	45	**33**

So again, we're just giving the cells what they need to repair themselves. It doesn't matter what's causing the inflammation. The inflammation will go away. If you've got chronic liver inflammation this program is for you too.

Chapter 50
Case Study #25

Reversing Multiple Sclerosis with Hyper-Nourishment

I have had a lot of success working with clients with Multiple Sclerosis or MS. The first person who came to me with MS back in 2016 was Nat. I met Nat for an online consultation using Skype. Nat was 41 years old at the time, and had been diagnosed with multiple sclerosis two years prior to our meeting. Prior to her diagnosis she was at her fittest, had a senior management job, and loved being a mother to her three sons. Her husband worked away a lot so she often felt like a single mother. She described her life as "crazy busy" but was managing to juggle everything she needed to do. The diagnosis came as a huge to her. When she first went to her doctor complaining about severe fatigue, she was referred to a neurologist. She said her neurologist told her "you will be right-most mums are tired". She told me "his view was let's wait till you can't walk before we do anything". She knew something was very wrong, and felt like a ticking time bomb.

Frustrated with her neurologist, she found another neurologist in Sydney who's clinic is purely for MS. She was great at validating her symptoms and explaining to her husband how sick she actually was. It felt good to be validated, that she really was sick and not lazy or the usual tired mother. While the validation felt better emotionally, it didn't help her disease get better. The medication she was on made her gain twelve pounds and caused her liver to be so inflamed that her liver tests looked like that of an alcoholic. It also suppressed her immune system which worried her, especially having three kids in school bringing home germs on a daily basis. When we met, she had been on the medicine for 12 months. Her doctor agreed it was not helping, and wanted to try stronger medication. At this point, after a year on a medicine with severe side effects, she felt worse than ever. Her nerve pain was higher than before, and her mobility was more limited than ever. She said at that point, she sometimes didn't even have enough energy to blink her eyes, and was spending much of her day in bed.

Desperate for a better way she went to a naturopath. The naturopath didn't have any treatments that helped her, but he gave her books and articles that led her to understand that a plant-based diet could make a big change in her symptoms. She contacted her friend who is a vegan athlete and asked her for resources, and her friend told her about me. She read up on me and started drinking green smoothies. Without any other changes, she suddenly had significantly more energy. She started contemplating going back to work after being unable to hold a job for two years because of her fatigue and pain. She made a Skype appointment to take her health to the next level, and was excited and hopeful for the first time in years.

She worked the program on her own after the consultation. Within three weeks her pain was completely gone. Four weeks later, May 6, 2016, she wrote me this message:

Hi Brooke how are you - amazing no doubt! Brooke I just want to give you an update on my journey since having that first initial Skype call with you back in April. After your call I have totally gone vegan and stuck to it. It is easy to stick to when results have been as amazing as they were for me!! I no longer suffer from that debilitating nerve pain or muscle fatigue!! I now can't remember the last time I had to spend days in bed unable to walk and only having the energy to move my eyes!!

I feel so empowered to have quality of life back and can't thank you enough for chatting with me in April and getting me motivated and started on my new health journey. You are the best THANK YOU SO MUCH xo. I checked in with Nat three years later, May 20, 2019, and she said this:

I am still going great... I am still ever so grateful to you!! From the moment I followed your protocol I haven't had that horrendous nerve pain back from all over my body!! It's incredible! I did introduce seafood back into my diet 10 months ago but mostly just plant-based still!! But to initially get rid of the extreme nerve pain I was experiencing I was a strict vegan as per your protocol for 9 months! Within 3 weeks noticed the difference! I couldn't believe it! I am still drug free and managing my MS symptoms beautifully. Only two things that flare it now are overheating and stress, so I just manage those two the best I can.

I am always referring people to your page!! Forever grateful to you!! And all the best with your new book! I will be sure to grab a copy! X Nat

Nat brings up a good point, that while you need to be very aggressive about the diet to reverse a disease, you don't have to stay strict to keep your health. Since she occasionally gets symptomatic with stress, she needs self-care to be a priority and make sure her diet is 100% plant-based and hyper-nourishing whenever stress is high to combat it the most effectively.

I've had multiple people in my 6 Week Rapid Recovery Group with Multiple Sclerosis. The first had "MS-Like" disease. She is a nurse with symptoms that her doctors told her were most likely caused by MS, but tests had not been able to confirm it yet. She had severe pain and exhaustion to where she had to stop working. After participating in the 6 Week Rapid Recovery Group, she reported she was "80% better". She said "my worst day now is like what my best day used to be." She felt so much better, she returned to her night shift nursing job after completing the short 6 week program.

Another group member had confirmed Multiple Sclerosis, and had a dramatic remission in her symptoms on a whole foods plant-based diet. She decided to join my 6 Week Rapid Recovery group to see if she could experience even greater benefits from taking her nutrition to the next level with hyper nourishment. She felt energetic and loved the program. Even better, when she received her next MRI, her most recent lesion was no longer visible on the MRI. The Radiologist could not explain the finding, and suggested that perhaps it was an "artifact." An artifact is when there is something on the MRI that was not actually present in the person, basically a screen error, like a scratch on a photograph. There was nothing to suggest it was an artifact when they saw the original MRI, they counted it as an MS lesion. However, without any medical explanation on how an MS lesion could actually disappear, the doctor concluded that the lesion just must not have been there to begin with, and it was instead a machine error. The lesion did not look like an artifact. Her improvement makes sense when you consider her anti-inflammatory nutrition program. His belief that a lesion wasn't real if it went away may sound bizarre, but this is not the first time doctors tried to explain away the results my clients experienced on this program. Rachel, someone you meet here in this book, reversed her Lupus and Sjogren's after four years of illness. When her laboratory tests were negative, one doctor tried to convince her she never had Lupus or Sjogren's to begin with. They are incurable diseases, so therefore if she got better she never had the diseases at all. When asked how she explained 4 years of positive tests, the doctor shrugged and said "lab error?" This doesn't explain the malar rashes, joint pain, dry eyes, dry mouth, miscarriages, and more she suffered with for years. She was so frustrated the doctor couldn't see how she healed.

While many doctors get excited when they witness their patients getting their health back on my program, many just refuse to acknowledge it, or dismiss it by saying, "keep doing whatever you're doing" without any curiosity about what they actually did. Even an intelligent person will go far to make up a story that lets them keep the same worldview they've always held. Thus, the bizarre but often repeated accusation, that since those diseases are incurable, you must never have had them to begin with, even though all the evidence points to the opposite.

In a recent group we had another client with multiple sclerosis who not only felt energetic and pain free, but she had a new MRI done at the completion of the group. Her MRI showed that the majority of her MS lesions on the MRI and shrunken considerably in size, and the newest lesion seen on the previous has MRI disappeared completely. She is electrified with hope and excitement about her future, knowing that she is healing, and doesn't have to live a life of illness and disability like her doctors had predicted. She is in control of her health now.

PART SIX
FAQ

Chapter 51
Frequently Asked Questions

Taking back your health is not just a dietary change – it's a lifestyle change. Here are the top questions I get asked regularly. I also do live question and answer sessions on a regular basis in our Facebook community (which you can join via the website SmoothieShred.com) and during my live online classes that I teach regularly. I announce my classes and Q&A sessions on social media, through my Instagram (#GoodbyeLupus) and Facebook page (Goodbye Lupus by Brooke Goldner MD).

1 - Is eating plant-based foods boring?

Foods taste better without being covered in all the junk we think makes them taste better. Plant-based, raw foods are delicious when you give them a chance to shine on their own instead of trying to hide their natural goodness under layers of butter, margarine, sour cream, etc. You'll notice food tastes different when it's free of all the extra fat and processed flavors. And I don't mean different bad; I mean different good. That being said, it takes about two to four weeks for people to stop craving foods they were addicted to, and appreciate the nuanced and delicious flavors in plant foods. So yes, at first, the food will likely taste boring, so you want to use self-care and fun in other areas of your life to entertain yourself, not unhealthy food!

2 - Will I have low energy if I only eat plant-based foods?

Low energy is an epidemic in our country. The issue is people do not have a caffeine deficiency. They have a nutrient deficiency. People who switch to a plant-based diet notice their energy levels are more consistent. Think of high-fiber and nutrient-heavy foods as the fire that burns for hours versus the low-fiber and nutrient-light foods extinguished in a flash. People who use the hyper-nourishing plan I teach, which is rich in raw foods, tell me they have more energy than they can ever remember.

3 - Can I get enough calcium eating a plant-based diet?

A diverse, plant-based diet is one of the best sources of calcium you'll find without the unhealthy effects of dairy. The best, most well-absorbed source of calcium for humans comes from leafy greens like broccoli and kale.

4 - Can carbs make me fat?

Carbohydrates have gotten a bad reputation, and undeservedly so. When most people think of carbs, they are envisioning processed carbohydrates like processed breads, pastas, and cakes. Realize though, all vegetables, beans, and fruits are sources of carbohydrates— good healthy carbohydrates! The key to superior health comes from eating a high carbohydrate diet. Carbs are your body's primary fuel source. They manage your heart rate, digestion, breathing, exercising, walking, and thinking. For healthy carbohydrates, the more you eat, the less fat you have.

5 - Are plant proteins complete proteins?

The old idea of needing to eat "complete proteins" has been disproven for many years. Plant proteins are as complete as you can find. The American Dietetic Association's position statement reads: "Plant sources of protein alone can provide adequate amounts of the essential and nonessential amino acids, assuming that dietary protein sources from plants are reasonably varied and that caloric intake suffices to meet energy needs. Whole grains, legumes, vegetables, seeds, and nuts all contain essential and nonessential amino acids."

6 - Can I get enough protein eating a plant-based diet?

You'd be surprised at the amount of protein you find in whole, natural plant-based foods. Spinach is 51 percent protein; mushrooms, 35 percent; beans, 26 percent; oatmeal, 16 percent; whole wheat pasta, 15 percent; corn, 12 percent; and potatoes, 11 percent. If you eat whole plant foods to fullness, you get enough protein for health. While physicians are inundated by patients suffering from diseases caused by eating too much meat, they will go their whole career without seeing one case of protein deficiency. The only way to have protein deficiency is to have a food deficit, basically to be starving.

7. What about caffeine?

If we have no energy, we often take something with caffeine in it to get ourselves through our days. This is a symptom of malnourishment since food should supply our energy, not caffeine. Also, people who are dependent on caffeine are usually much more fatigued, as they over-stimulate their nervous system and end up more tired in the long run. That said, people have done fine on my programs having 1 cup of coffee a day, as long as there is no sugar or dairy in it. A better choice is green tea, which has some anti-inflammatory properties. A cup of green tea a day is okay. Also, be cautious about suddenly stopping caffeine use. Caffeine is a laxative and often times when people suddenly stop caffeine and then load up on fiber in my program, they get severely constipated. A slow taper is a better way to kick the caffeine habit.

8. What about alcohol?

Alcohol is inflammatory and will slow down or undo your healing. When you are healthy, it is okay to have a glass of alcohol occasionally; it will spike inflammation but a healthy body can recover from that quickly. While you are trying to reverse your disease, it's best to avoid it so your body can focus itself on recovery.

9. What about gluten?

Gluten is found in wheat, rye, barley, and many processed foods. You will find it in foods like traditional breads and pasta. I believe that most people who believe they have gluten sensitivity are reacting to processed grains. If you have a diagnosed sensitivity to gluten, it's best to avoid it. Also, it has been suggested that 40% or more people with autoimmune diseases also have some sensitivity to gluten. Therefore, for a faster recovery, it's best to avoid it. Note that gluten-containing foods are not part of the rapid recovery plan. If you would like to add whole unprocessed grains but are worried about sensitivity, try going off gluten-containing products for a few weeks and then reintroduce them when you are feeling better. Again, it is unnecessary to consume grains for this healing protocol. I have not found it to have healing properties and consider it a health-maintenance food rather than a healing food.

10. Do I need any supplements?

This is a whole food approach to healing, so no other vitamins are required to nourish your cells and begin the healing process. The newest research shows that many people suffer from a dysfunctional gut from the effects of meat, dairy, and processed foods on their healthy bacteria and gut wall. That said, here are the supplements that I most often recommend:

1. Probiotics: It is often helpful to add a high-grade probiotic during the first couple months of changing your diet, which helps digestion and maximize the benefits from eating well.
2. Vitamin D3: Most people I encounter are deficient in D and need to take D3 as a replacement. If you are low in D vitamins, you will have a slower recovery since it is a necessary component of immune function. The best thing to do is ask for a blood test to check your vitamin D levels.
3. Vitamin B12: B12 is normally derived from bacteria that live in fecal matter.[26] You have a huge supply of B12 in your gut bacteria right now, but you don't have access to it.[27] When people ate vegetables from the ground that was recently fertilized by animals passing through and snacking on the same plant, they received B12 from the dirty plant. Nowadays, animals are kept far away from our crops, and everything is "triple-washed", so we don't get the same amount of B12 from plants that we used to. People who eat meat regularly eat food that is contaminated by fecal matter, because of fecal contamination in animal products.[28,29] When you stop eating animals, you eat fewer feces, and therefore less B12. B12 can be supplemented with fortified foods like fortified nutritional yeast or B12 supplements. How much you need of either depends on your levels, so the best thing you can do is have your doctor test your B12 levels so he or she can recommend how to replace it if you need to. Someone with normal levels can usually just use a supplement once or twice a week or use fortified foods. Someone with a deficiency needs to take it daily. If oral replacement doesn't work, you might have a problem with oral absorption (more common in elderly adults) and need to take the intramuscular injections instead.

Message for the reader from Dr. Goldner

Thank you so much for purchasing and reading this book. My greatest desire is to inspire and educate people to take back their health and live their best life. I hope reading this truly changes your life, bringing you immense health and happiness.

If you need more help and support to reach your health goals, I do as much as I can to help people for free. I frequently put on online webinar classes, make numerous YouTube videos, and social media posts to educate and inspire others to make the best choices and live the best life possible.

To get access to my free content, upcoming events where you can see me speak, or to learn more about how I can personally help you, through consultations or to join my next 6 Week Rapid Recovery Group, go to

http://GoodbyeAutoimmuneDisease.com

I wish you amazing health and joy!

Brooke Goldner, M.D.

CITATIONS

1. Saeed Alshahrani, Gary Fraser, Joan Sabaté, Raymond Knutsen, David Shavlik, Andrew Mashchak, Jan Lloren, Michael Orlich. Red and Processed Meat and Mortality in a Low Meat Intake Population. Nutrients, 2019; 11 (3): 622 DOI: 10.3390/nu11030622

2. C Mary Schooling, Milk & Mortality, BMJ 2014;349:g6205

3. Rueda-Clausen CF1, Silva FA, Lindarte MA, Villa-Roel C, Gomez E, Gutierrez R, Cure-Cure C, López-Jaramillo P. Olive, soybean and palm oils intake have a similar acute detrimental effect over the endothelial function in healthy young subjects. Nutr Metab Cardiovasc Dis. 2007 Jan;17(1):50-7. Epub 2006 Mar 20.

4. J Obes. Anti-Inflammatory Nutrition as a Pharmacological Approach to Treat Obesity 2011; 2011: 431985.

5. Hu Y1, Costenbader KH1, Gao X1, Al-Daabil M1, Sparks JA1, Solomon DH1, Hu FB1, Karlson EW1, Lu B1, Sugar-sweetened soda consumption and risk of developing rheumatoid arthritis in women, Am J Clin Nutr. 2014 Sep;100(3):959-67.

6. Baer DJ1, Judd JT, Clevidence BA, Tracy RP. Dietary fatty acids affect plasma markers of inflammation in healthy men fed controlled diets: a randomized crossover study. Am J Clin Nutr. 2004 Jun;79(6):969-73.

7. Han SN1, Leka LS, Lichtenstein AH, Ausman LM, Schaefer EJ, Meydani SN. Effect of hydrogenated and saturated, relative to polyunsaturated, fat on immune and inflammatory responses of adults with moderate hypercholesterolemia. J Lipid Res. 2002 Mar;43(3):445-52.

8. Bendsen NT1, Stender S, Szecsi PB, Pedersen SB, Basu S, Hellgren LI, Newman JW, Larsen TM, Haugaard SB, Astrup A.Effect of industrially produced trans fat on markers of systemic inflammation: evidence from a randomized trial in women. J Lipid Res. 2011 Oct;52(10):1821-8. doi: 10.1194/jlr.M014738. Epub 2011 Jul 27.

9. Lopez-Garcia E1, Schulze MB, Meigs JB, Manson JE, Rifai N, Stampfer MJ, Willett WC, Hu FB. Consumption of trans fatty acids is related to

plasma biomarkers of inflammation and endothelial dysfunction. J Nutr. 2005 Mar;135(3):562-6.

10. Maria Alessandra Gammone,1,* Graziano Riccioni,1,2 Gaspare Parrinello,3 and Nicolantonio D'Orazio. Omega-3 Polyunsaturated Fatty Acids: Benefits and Endpoints in Sport. Nutrients. 2019 Jan; 11(1): 46.

11. Wall R., Ross R.P., Fitzgerald G.F., Stanton C. Fatty acids from fish: The anti-inflammatory potential of long-chain omega-3 fatty acids. Nutr. Rev. 2010;68:280–289. doi: 10.1111/j.1753-4887.2010.00287.x. [PubMed] [CrossRef] [Google Scholar].

12. Lunn J., Theobald H. The health effects of dietary unsaturated fatty acids. Nutr. Bull. 2006;31:178–224. doi: 10.1111/j.1467-3010.2006.00571.x. [CrossRef] [Google Scholar]

13. Michail, M., Giannou, K., When did coloring books become mindful? Exploring the effectiveness of a novel method of mindfulness - guided instructions for coloring books to increase mindfulness and decrease anxiety. Front Psychol. 2018; 9: 56.

14. Yun-Zi Liu, Yun-Xia Wang, and Chun-Lei Jiang,, Inflammation: The Common Pathway of Stress-Related Diseases. Front Hum Neurosci. 2017; 11: 316.

15. Andrew H. Miller,, Charles L. Raison. The role of inflammation in depression: from evolutionary imperative to modern treatment target. Nat Rev Immunol. 2016 Jan; 16(1): 22–34.

16. N Vogelzangs, A T F Beekman,P de Jonge, B W J H Penninx. Anxiety disorders and inflammation in a large adult cohort. Transl Psychiatry. 2013 Apr; 3(4): e249.

17. Goran Medic, Micheline Wille, Michiel EH Hemels. Short- and long-term health consequences of sleep disruption. Nat Sci Sleep. 2017; 9: 151–161.

18. Watson NF, Badr MS, Belenky G, Bliwise DL, Buxton OM, Buysse D, Dinges DF, Gangwisch J, Grandner MA, Kushida C, Malhotra RK, Martin JL, Patel SR, Quan SF, Tasali E. Joint Consensus Statement of the American Academy of Sleep Medicine and Sleep Research Society on the

Recommended Amount of Sleep for a Healthy Adult: Methodology and Discussion. Sleep. 2015 Aug 1; 38(8):1161-83.

19. Olesen J, Gustavsson A, Svensson M, Wittchen HU, Jönsson B, CDBE2010 The economic cost of brain disorders in Europe. European Brain Council. Eur J Neurol. 2012 Jan; 19(1):155-62.

20. A.N. Perry, C. Westenbroek, J.B. Becker. The Development of a Preference for Cocaine over Food Identifies Individual Rats with Addiction-Like BehaviorsPLoS One. 2013; 8(11): e79465.

21. Huan Song, MD, PhD1,2; Fang Fang, MD, PhD2; Gunnar Tomasson, MD, PhD3,4,5; et al Filip K. Arnberg, PhD6,7; David Mataix-Cols, PhD8,9; Lorena Fernández de la Cruz, PhD8; Catarina Almqvist, MD, PhD2,10; Katja Fall, MD, PhD11,12; Unnur A. Valdimarsdóttir, PhD1,2,13 , Association of Stress-Related Disorders With Subsequent Autoimmune Disease. JAMA. 2018;319(23):2388-2400. doi:10.1001/jama.2018.7028

22. Helland IB1, Smith L, Saarem K, Saugstad OD, Drevon CA., Maternal supplementation with very-long-chain n-3 fatty acids during pregnancy and lactation augments children's IQ at 4 years of age. Pediatrics. 2003 Jan;111(1):e39-44.

23. Jensen CL1., Effects of n-3 fatty acids during pregnancy and lactation., Am J Clin Nutr. 2006 Jun;83(6 Suppl):1452S-1457S.

24. Marpaung, B., 220 Relationship between increased levels of anti-dsdna with clinical symptoms in patients with SLE. Poster Session, SLE Organ manifestations: clinical and pathogenesis

25. Barnard, N., Cohen, J., Jenkins, D., Turner-McGrievy, G., Gloede, L., Green, A., and Ferdowsian, H., A low-fat vegan diet and a conventional diabetes diet in the treatment of type 2 diabetes: a randomized, controlled, 74-wk clinical trial. Am J Clin Nutr. 2009 May; 89(5): 1588S–1596S.

26. F. O'Leary, S. Samman. Vitamin B12 in Health and Disease. Nutrients. 2010 Mar; 2(3): 299–316.

27. P.H. Degnan, M.E. Taga, A.L. Goodman. Vitamin B12 as a modulator of gut microbial ecology. Cell Metab. 2014 Nov 4; 20(5): 769–778.

28. U. Lyhs, I. Ikonen, T. Pohjanvirta, K. Raninen, P. Perko-Mäkelä, S. Pelkonen Extraintestinal pathogenic Escherichia coli in poultry meat products on the Finnish retail market. *Acta Veterinaria Scandinavica* **volume 54**, 64 (2012)

29. J. Hyun Kim, S.J. Hur, D. Gyun Yim Monitoring of Microbial Contaminants of Beef, Pork, and Chicken in HACCP Implemented Meat Processing Plants of Korea Korean J Food Sci Anim Resour. 2018 Apr; 38(2): 282–290.

30. G. C. Curhan, MD, ScD. Epidemiology of Stone Disease. Urol Clin North Am. 2007 Aug; 34(3): 287–293.

31. Mathew D. Sorensen, MD, MS, Ryan S. Hsi, MD, Thomas Chi, MD, Nawar Shara, MS, PhD, Jean Wactawski-Wende, PhD, Arnold J. Kahn, PhD, Hong Wang, MD, MS, Lifang Hou, MD, PhD, and Marshall L. Stoller, MD. Dietary Intake of Fiber, Fruit, and Vegetables Decrease the Risk of Incident Kidney Stones in Women: A Women's Health Initiative (WHI) Report. J Urol. 2014 Dec; 192(6): 1694–1699.

32. Khneizer G, Al-Taee A, Mallick MS, Bastani B. Chronic dietary oxalate nephropathy after intensive dietary weight loss regimen. J Nephropathol. 2017 Jul;6(3):126-129. doi: 10.15171/jnp.2017.21.

33. akkapati S, D'Agati VD, Balsam L. "Green Smoothie Cleanse" Causing Acute Oxalate Nephropathy. Am J Kidney Dis. 2018 Feb;71(2):281-286. doi:10.1053/j.ajkd.2017.08.002.